Human Services Integration

Human Services Integration

Michael J. Austin, PhD
Editor

Routledge
Taylor & Francis Group
NEW YORK AND LONDON

Human Services Integration has also been published as *Administration in Social Work*, Volume 21, Numbers 3/4 1997.

First published 1997 by The Haworth Press, Inc.

This edition published 2013 by Routledge
605 Third Avenue, New York, NY 10017
2 Park Square, Milton Park, Abingdon, Oxon OX14 4RN

Routledge is an imprint of the Taylor & Francis Group, an informa business

Cover design by Thomas J. Mayshock Jr.

Library of Congress Cataloging-in-Publication Data

Human services integration / Michael J. Austin, editor.
p. cm.
"Has also been published as Administration in social work, volume 21, numbers 3/4 1997"–T.p. verso.
Includes bibliographical references and index.
ISBN 0-7890-0353-8 (alk. paper)
1. Human services–United States. 2. Social service–United States. 3. Community organizations–United States. I. Austin, Michael J.
HV91.H773 1997
361.973–dc21 97-37551
CIP

ISBN13 : 978-0-7890-0353-9 (hbk)

Human Services Integration

CONTENTS

ABOUT THE EDITOR

Michael J. Austin, PhD, ACSW, is Professor in the School of Social Welfare at the University of California at Berkeley. The former Dean of the University of Pennsylvania School of Social Work, he teaches graduate students in the area of administration and community planning. During the last 25 years, he has also taught at Florida State University and the University of Washington. Prior to beginning his academic career, he served as a management consultant for the National Institute of Mental Health and as a planner for United Way Planning Agencies in California. He also served as a management consultant to the Philadelphia Department of Human Services, the Florida Department of Health and Rehabilitation Services, and numerous other local, state, and national agencies. Currently, he serves as a consultant to the Bay Area Social Services Consortium, a twelve county and four university partnership related to policy, research, and training. He is the author of three books related to child welfare: *Supervisory Management for the Human Services* (Prentice Hall), *Managing Staff Development Programs in Human Service Agencies* (Nelson-Hall), and *Managing Human Service Personnel* (Sage). He has also written 12 books in the area of human service administration and 40 professional articles.

Service Integration: Introduction

Michael J. Austin, PhD

The integration of human services has come to acquire over the past two decades many different meanings. For some, it means doing a better job of coordinating across human service programs and organizations. For others, it involves the physical co-location of services networked together. For still others, service integration refers to the fundamental restructuring of human service organizations to improve service delivery at the neighborhood, community, county, and regional levels.

In addition to addressing the multiple meanings of service integration, this volume represents a small but important effort to take a look at some lessons learned. For newcomers to the concept of service integration, as well as for the old-timers who may have forgotten, the articles by Hassett and Austin, and by Adams and Nelson, provide an important overview. For those interested in seeing how the vision of service integration in different communities gets translated into the realities of everyday life, the case studies by Armstrong and Minicucci provide lessons about collaboration as well as resistance to change. For those interested in finding ways to assess the processes of service integration and service coordination, the articles by O'Looney and by Harbert, Finnegan, and Tyler represent current research findings and challenges. And finally, for those interested in exploring social science theory relevant to service integration, the article by Halley, discusses the potential of boundary-spanning theory.

Each of the articles contributes to the knowledge base of service in-

Michael J. Austin is Professor, School of Social Welfare, University of California at Berkeley, Berkeley, CA 94720.

[Haworth co-indexing entry note]: "Service Integration: Introduction." Austin, Michael J. Co-published simultaneously in *Administration in Social Work* (The Haworth Press, Inc.) Vol. 21, No. 3/4, 1997, pp. 1-7; and: *Human Services Integration* (ed: Michael J. Austin) The Haworth Press, Inc., 1997, pp. 1-7. Single or multiple copies of this article are available for a fee from The Haworth Document Delivery Service [1-800-342-9678, 9:00 a.m. - 5:00 p.m. (EST). E-mail address: getinfo@haworth.com].

tegration. They also help to frame an evolving research agenda for future inquiry such as: Why is it so difficult to institutionalize, over time, service integration innovations into existing human service systems? Why is the measuring of service integration so difficult? How can the resistance to new forms of service delivery practice be better understood? What is the impact of the culture of organizations and the environment of local communities upon service integration initiatives? How could social science theory more directly inform the practice of service integration? Readers of this book will, no doubt, identify other questions worthy of further investigation.

One of the more intriguing issues emerging from this set of articles involves the connection between service integration and a possible vision of a human service system in the 21st century. A vision of an ideal human service system is often more implicit than explicit in much of the service integration literature. In an effort to articulate a vision, a group of county social and human service directors, deans of schools of social work, and local foundation representatives in Northern California (Bay Area Social Services Consortium) crafted a vision statement to guide their efforts in transforming their organizations. Such a vision takes on new importance in the light of welfare reform and the opportunity to use block grants to reconfigure human service delivery systems. An excerpt of the BASSC statement, "Human Services–2000," is noted below (Bay Area Social Service Consortium, "Human Services–2000" Berkeley, CA: University of California, School of Social Welfare, 1994).

> In the 21st century, members of the Bay Area Social Services Consortium (BASSC) envision a community service system that will serve all families in need. As an equal opportunity service provider, it will serve a neighborhood-based constituency whereby the service users are also the owners of the service. It will provide a universal service, not a residual one; that is, it will serve all people who do not have an intact or sufficiently strong personal support system (nuclear or extended family) to help them meet their basic needs for survival and growth. This philosophy is based on a prevention model of services to families and children that seeks to educate consumers to utilize available service supports and empowers them by fostering self-sufficiency. Since the goal of a prevention-oriented system is to reach all those in need, the outcome of the service system is measured on the basis of community health and social supports, not by the impact of services on individuals.
>
> The activities of the human service system will be located in a

specially designed neighborhood community center. Those who enter the center will be greeted by a welcoming environment that promotes accessibility and a sense of entitlement as a citizen, where people are valued for their individuality and diversity. The scale of the center is small and the sense of neighborhood ownership is large. The center will be based on a community approach to problem-solving, rather than an individualistic one. State and county governments will be less visible in the center and will not be the exclusive means for delivering services. The neighborhood center, whether it is urban or rural, will be built and maintained in much the same way and spirit that a barn is raised collectively in rural farm country.

In addition to treating community members fairly, the core values of the center's activities will be linked to the use of 'behind the scenes' universal governmental programs that maximize the accumulation of social and financial resources to preserve families. The key values are to minimize governmental regulation, to avoid notions of 'less-than-humane' subsistence levels of living, and to guarantee access to a minimal level of care and support in times of need. Services will be structured on a non-categorical approach to people in need because the center will operate on the belief that individuals and neighborhoods have the capacity to change and improve over time. All services will reflect a commitment to racial and cultural diversity. The center will operate on a shared sense of equal opportunity and a commitment to create a greater good for all. The center services will be built upon a substantial commitment to the promotion of employment and economic self-sufficiency and the provision of role models for working people and for youths. Public assistance will be viewed as temporary entitlement between jobs and/or childbirth and will be linked to child care support services.

The neighborhood service center will be known for its comprehensive array of interdisciplinary services for children, families, adults, and senior citizens. It will operate as a well-managed comprehensive human service agency offering effective professional and volunteer services. The center will reflect a sense of community pride in the health and welfare of its families and residents. It will be a responsive, caring and helpful organization that respects people; it will provide culturally relevant neighborhood services based on prevention and early intervention. The welfare of children and the aged will be incorporated into an overall plan for family support to assist people in making life better for themselves. Neighborhood residents will participate as both recipients of services and owners of services through a representative board of directors. The outcomes of service delivery will be assessed regularly in order to determine unmet needs, foster ownership, and maximize the partnership between service providers and service recipients.

Two key values underlie the philosophy imbedded in the vision statement. The first is community. It has become abundantly clear that meeting the needs of individuals and families requires a collaborative community approach. Service fragmentation and legislated mandates leading to turf battles can no longer be tolerated. A community approach means professionals and consumers work together as partners in managing the human services system. This means working with existing community institutions (e.g., schools, courts, correctional services, and churches). It means connecting the local/regional economic marketplace with the human service marketplace (e.g., housing, food, clothing, and jobs). And it means working under new federal policies to invest in families through a common funding stream in order to support citizens in need. As the old African proverb suggests, 'It takes a whole village to raise a child.'

The second key value is tangible outcomes of community betterment. This value moves beyond measuring outcome at the individual level and focuses on how well a neighborhood is doing. Criteria for assessment include: community responses to changing neighborhood demographics; the degree of involvement of extended families in service programs which utilize ethnically-sensitive practice; the degree to which temporary family supports are complemented by long-term supports; the extent of citizen participation; the extent to which professionals work together in interdisciplinary practice; the degree to which neighborhood systems advocate for the total community; and the extent to which the needs of middle-class families are integrated with those of low-income families.

The following major service delivery principles that underlie the framework of the BASSC vision statement are clustered into three major categories:

- *Principles of Resource Distribution*
  - Fairness and Equity
  - Adequacy of Income/Economic Support
  - Equality of Access and Opportunity

- *Principles of Decision-Making and Authority*
  - A Community Approach to Problem-Solving
  - Consumer Ownership
  - A Decentralized Neighborhood-Based Service Delivery System

- *Principles of Service Design and Delivery*
  - Proactive Prevention-Oriented Services
  - A Deep Commitment to Racial and Cultural Diversity
  - Comprehensive and Non-Categorical Services
  - Universal Federal Family Investment Policies

FACILITATING THE ADOPTION AND IMPLEMENTATION OF THE VISION

There are significant administrative challenges to helping local communities develop their own approach to assisting children, families, and adults. These include: fostering community leadership; supporting staff autonomy and creativity; transferring authority and responsibility from state and county government to local units; and developing safeguards to assure accountability in the use of public funds.

Another administrative challenge is to design inter-agency mechanisms that will assist local community service centers to link with key institutions in the areas of job training, economic development, local taxing authority, public education, and environmental monitoring. The relationship between economic development and social development needs to be fully described, understood, and modified at the local level. Similarly, the full impact of human service expenditures on a local economy needs to be assessed and converted into an investment strategy that will provide supports throughout the life cycle for people in need. Addressing these challenges requires shifting from old ways to new ways of managing the process of change.

When it comes to implementing a vision within the context of local government and neighborhoods, the following realities need to be clearly understood and integrated by those who assume key social service agency leadership roles in managing change in the direction of a new vision:

I. Organizational Self-Assessment

- Helping all parties identify the current structures and processes that are not working is a way to link the present with the future.
- Assessing the agency's culture and climate at all levels requires the careful collection and understanding of staff frustrations and difficulties, especially with respect to the leadership capacities of management staff.

- Recognizing that it is critical to get one's own agency in order prior to, or in conjunction with, exploring the potentials for new service structures at the community and neighborhood levels.

II. Planning

- Developing a vision statement which emerges out of, or precedes, the development and implementation of a strategic plan.
- Investing in planning processes by involving internal and external stakeholders at all levels of deliberation is key to implementing a vision.

III. Managing Change

- Structuring a senior team to guide the change process is critical and can take the form of a special assistant to the director (guiding and monitoring systems serving as the eyes and ears of the director), a director of staff development (designing and implementing staff retreats and training sessions), and a quality assurance director (redesigning information systems to facilitate decision-making and service outcome evaluation).
- Recognizing that humanizing the workplace is an essential ingredient of the change process (e.g., agency holiday parties, picnics, receptions) as well as ongoing written communications (agency newsletter, staff memos recognizing special efforts).
- Encountering resistance requires patience and strategic thinking in order to work around and/or isolate resistors and then welcome them into the fold when the realization strikes that the train of change has left the station and it is possible to still get on board.
- Recognizing that the greatest source of creative new ideas can be line staff if they are encouraged to communicate in writing, and informally, with the agency director and protected by the director with regard to any repercussions for bypassing the chain of command.
- Implementing a vision requires a long time horizon, minimum of five years.

IV. Administrative Leadership

- Changing the role of management from reactive, controlling behaviors to proactive, facilitating behaviors (coach, mentor, teacher) up and down the management hierarchy is essential in order to help others assess progress made toward achieving the vision.

- Understanding that management by walking around and talking with all levels of staff in their work areas every 3-6 months can be a critical element for the agency director to keep track of the pulse of the change process.
- Keeping the governing board and the Board of Supervisors apprised of progress towards the vision is essential and made easier if the Board has appointed a human services oversight council focused primarily on developing and implementing a strategic plan for the agency.
- Realizing that all significant progress in managing change in pursuit of a new vision can be enhanced by the use of outside consultants to assist with guiding the process, training the participants, facilitating retreats on highly charged topics, and providing an external view of complex issues.

This BASSC Vision Statement raises many questions regarding service integration. How is citizen participation connected with service integration? Preliminary answers are noted in the North Richmond neighborhood which Armstrong describes. How do administrators monitor service integration efforts? O'Looney seeks to address this question as it emerged in Georgia. And finally, how do the principles of decision-making interact with the principles of resource distribution and service delivery?

As with all special publications, it is hoped that the ideas brought together in this one volume will provide administrators, researchers, and students with much food for thought as service integration takes on new meaning in this era of welfare reform.

Service Integration: Something Old and Something New

Seth Hassett, MSW
Michael J. Austin, PhD

SUMMARY. The authors trace the definition and challenges of "service integration," variously known over time as "collaboration," "coordination," "human services integration," and "one-stop shopping." While the common use of service integration terminology currently may seem to indicate a consensus in favor of a broad systemic reform, motivations and expectations for service integration differ significantly among different players in the service system. The authors conclude that service integration cannot be defined by a particular service model or outcome, but instead should be conceived of as an ongoing reform process. This process, when well-designed and implemented with long-term vision, can reduce duplication, strengthen communities, and improve client outcomes. *[Article copies available for a fee from The Haworth Document Delivery Service: 1-800-342-9678. E-mail address: getinfo@haworth.com]*

Service Integration (SI) efforts fall under a variety of labels including "collaboration," "coordination," "human services integration," "one-stop shopping" and many others. While these labels may signify different levels of intensity or differing focus, they all refer to efforts to reduce or

---

Seth Hassett is a Public Health Analyst, Center for Mental Health Services, Substance Abuse and Mental Health Administration, Washington, DC. Michael J. Austin is Professor, School of Social Welfare, University of California at Berkeley, Berkeley, CA 94720.

[Haworth co-indexing entry note]: "Service Integration: Something Old and Something New." Hassett, Seth, and Michael J. Austin. Co-published simultaneously in *Administration in Social Work* (The Haworth Press, Inc.) Vol. 21, No. 3/4, 1997, pp. 9-29; and: *Human Services Integration* (ed: Michael J. Austin) The Haworth Press, Inc., 1997, pp. 9-29. Single or multiple copies of this article are available for a fee from The Haworth Document Delivery Service [1-800-342-9678, 9:00 a.m. - 5:00 p.m. (EST). E-mail address: getinfo@haworth.com].

eliminate divisions or boundaries between categorically defined and provided services. Efforts at service integration can take place within a single organization providing multiple services or between separate organizations and agencies providing related services. Some of the challenges related to service integration will be considered following a brief exploration of the historical developments behind current interest in the issue.

THE EMERGENCE OF SERVICE INTEGRATION

The term "service integration" came into common use within the human service system during the late 1960s and early 1970s, but concerns over coordinating charitable or public services date back much further. For example, Lynn (1980) traces some of the service integration themes as far back as the Civil War. By the turn of the 20th century, state and local governments were called upon to develop policies to address major social needs associated with large numbers of war victims, the emancipation of slaves, an influx of immigrants, accelerated industrialization and recurring economic depressions.

Through the first decades of the 20th century, the bulk of services to the poor were carried out through private charitable organizations with government at all levels assuming a very limited role (Soler & Shauffer, 1990). Within the private charitable sector, however, efforts were made to address multiple needs in an integrated manner. For example, neighborhood-based settlement houses provided a variety of services to children and families in one location, while progressive reformers associated with the settlement houses sought to address the root causes of poverty (Soler & Shauffer, 1990; Lynn, 1980).

The social, economic, and political upheavals of the Great Depression created increased public acceptance in the 1930s for a larger state and federal role in the social welfare system. The Social Security Act of 1935 instituted federal grants-in-aid for dependent children, the blind and aged, as well as programs for crippled children, maternal and child health, child welfare and public health. Grants were targeted toward specific population groups based on defined categories of need, thereby requiring investigation of eligibility for government assistance. While this 1935 landmark legislation has been amended twenty times, the definitions of client need set the precedent for growth in categorical human service programs in the 1960s and beyond.

The first major efforts at services integration were aimed at coordinating the administration of programs at local levels. For example, the Model Cities program required many cities to become involved for the first time in efforts to bring together a wide range of social services and to foster citizen involvement subjecting local officials to new political controversy and criticism (Soler & Shauffer, citing Yessian & Lang in *The Quest for Human Services Integration as Reflected in HEW*, 1981).

In the 1970s, services integration was envisioned and attempted on a grander scale. Elliot Richardson, Secretary of Health, Education and Welfare (HEW) under President Nixon, promoted an ambitious agenda for services integration, including research and demonstration projects, technical assistance efforts, and organizational reforms (Kusserow, 1991). Some aspects of the reform agenda, proposed in the ill-fated 1972 Allied Services Act, would have given state and local elected officials more latitude in how federal funds for the human services were spent (Lynn, 1980). However, in 1972 the federal government launched ten technical assistance projects and 35 research and demonstration projects. Called SITO (Services Integration Targets of Opportunity), the projects sought comprehensive service delivery at the state and local level through interagency program linkages in the areas of fiscal, personnel, planning and programming, administrative support, core services and case coordination (Family Impact Seminar, 1991; Gardner, 1976; Horton et al., 1976; John, 1977).

Despite the promise of innovative service integration, by the mid-1970s, many of the projects were not seen as successful and were discontinued. According to Soler and Shauffer, SITO "failed because of its architects limited understanding of the communities it was designed to serve" (Soler & Shauffer, 1990). The service integration initiatives sought to implement a "grand design" of an integrated service system to meet the needs of persons and families at risk. Few such designs could be built quickly enough to satisfy all the interested parties. Secondly, the expectation of many supporters was that service integration would result in cost savings, and when most projects failed to show such savings within a few years, many supporters lost interest. Thirdly, while the impetus for service integration came largely from the top levels of federal and local governments, there was significant staff resistance at the service delivery levels where professionals in expanding categorical services often had little incentive to cooperate and integrate services. And finally, evaluative studies concluded that most SITO projects were expensive and had failed to meet their major objectives (John, 1977). The demise of these projects signaled the end of the major "top-down" push for service integration. By the early 1980s, the attention of federal, state, and local human service administrators was diverted from innovative initiatives to protecting their programs in an era of massive cutbacks and tightening budgets.

Yet, as Agranoff (1991) states, reports of the demise of service integration were premature since many of the projects continued to operate in some form at state and local levels. By the late 1980s, service integration had reemerged as a focus of reform efforts. "Buzz words" such as "collaboration," "coordination," "one-stop shopping" and "seamless service provision" came into increasing use in the human service community over a decade after federal, state, and local attention had been diverted by cutbacks. However, this new movement was not simply a rebirth of earlier efforts since it differed significantly from the earlier "grand design" system-oriented efforts and focused more on targeting service integration toward a more modest set of problems or populations (Agranoff & Pattakos, 1979). While this service-oriented approach to service integration may be more modest in scope than earlier system-oriented strategies, the targeted approach may be more realistic, effective, and sustainable (U.S. General Accounting Office, 1992). The Family Impact Seminar (1991) cites five features that distinguish the current service integration movement from earlier efforts and make it a potentially more significant change effort:

1. *Greater Breadth and Depth*. Interest and activity is occurring in every human service sector. Education is interested for the first time in taking active role.
2. *Multi-Level*. Reforms are being initiated simultaneously from top down and bottom up.
3. *New Technology*. Rapidly evolving new computer technology creates the potential for computerized one-stop applications and eligibility determinations that were not previously possible.
4. *Budget Tightening*. Service integration is occurring at a time of serious fiscal stringency at all levels of government. Therefore the emphasis on service integration as a route to reducing costs is even more intense.
5. *Family-Focus*. The current reform movement is more clearly focused than earlier service integration efforts on viewing the family as a unit of service and developing new technologies and approaches for implementing family-centered services. (p. 10)

LESSONS LEARNED AND UNRESOLVED CHALLENGES

While these five features may make the current service integration movement more sustainable and effective than earlier efforts, there are still many pitfalls on the road to reform. Lessons can be learned from the efforts of the 1960s and 1970s such as the importance of long-term vision, the need for realistic expectations and clearly defined achievable objectives, and the need for staff and community "buy-in" at all levels. The service integration movement includes many models that attempt to account for these issues, but many underlying issues are unresolved. Among these issues are those of conflicting visions and motivations for reform, fragmented service integration efforts, centralized versus decentralized administration, new staff roles, confidentiality issues, the need for agency sacrifice.

While the common use of service integration terminology may seem to indicate a consensus in favor of broad systemic reform, motivations and expectations for service integration, in fact, differ significantly among different players in the service system. For instance, client advocates generally view service integration projects as a means for providing more comprehensive and seamless services to individuals and families with complex needs. Their vision of an integrated service system often involves filling gaps in services to needy populations. Filling these service gaps often involves new–and sometimes costly–services such as case management, transportation, child care services, job training, and increased health benefits. At the same time, some administrators and elected officials focus on service integration primarily as a means of providing existing services more efficiently. In times of budget cutbacks, service integration may be viewed as a means for preserving existing services by eliminating duplication and waste.

These two visions–that of SI as a means toward comprehensive services and that of SI as a means toward more efficient provision of services–are not necessarily mutually exclusive, but as the struggles of the 1960s and 1970s demonstrate, they should not be expected to reconcile themselves naturally. Failure to develop consensus on the purposes for service integration efforts at the administrative, staff, and community levels will severely hinder efforts to set achievable goals and objectives and secure cooperation at all levels. It should be clear at the outset that eliminating duplication and waste can free up resources for providing additional needed services, but only if any savings are reallocated within the human services system.

As efforts to integrate services become more popular, demonstration projects are proliferating in many state and county systems. The diversity of projects allows planning coalitions to tailor their processes toward the specific needs of targeted communities or population groups. In many instances, however, integrated services projects are not adequately coordinated with one another (Kahn & Kamerman, 1992). For instance, a variety of computer information systems may be developed at once, each with a vision for expansion throughout the broader service system. Without communication and coordination between parallel developments, the promise of computerized one-stop applications and eligibility determinations may be lost as different programs become committed to costly and possibly incompatible systems.

Fragmented service integration efforts may occur within relatively small communities, especially those with complex problems and needs. Due to the compelling nature of community needs, several community planning efforts may be developed simultaneously. Through coordinated communication and linkages, these parallel planning efforts can strengthen one another, but turf disputes can also arise, just as they can between separate agencies and professional groups.

While the concept of services integration does not specify either a centralized or decentralized model, the general thrust of most current service integration efforts is toward a more decentralized system of neighborhood-based services. While theoretically attractive, this decentralized approach must be undertaken carefully in order to avoid greater fragmentation and inequity throughout the larger service system. As local communities assume greater fiscal and administrative responsibility for human services, those communities with more resources may be in a better position to take advantage of new opportunities. While funding may be targeted toward disadvantaged communities, members of these communities may not be sufficiently prepared to advocate for their needs within the larger service system.

As regulations become less universal and standardized, some progressive communities may move to provide a comprehensive range of services to all their residents while others may seek to cut services or may provide services only to the most vocal or active elements of their communities. As the Model Cities projects demonstrated, increased decision-making autonomy can put an intolerable strain on local governments as political pressure mounts from various neighborhood groups, all with compelling arguments for their needs. This pressure is likely to be even more intense if, as is often the case, decentralization places additional responsibilities on local governments while placing severe restrictions on how funds can be spent. To be successful, service integration at local levels will require a difficult balance of more flexible financing approaches along with safeguards to assure attention to the needs of disadvantaged populations and communities.

Many integrated service models include redefinitions of professional roles, with greater autonomy and flexibility at the direct service level. While this autonomy is empowering to motivated professionals, it assumes a level of competency that cannot always be guaranteed. New roles and responsibilities may put additional pressures and unrealistic expectations on line staff. Without clear eligibility guidelines for who to serve, and with limited resources available, staff may be forced to refuse services to needy individuals and families based on professional judgment. Some workers accustomed to dealing with a narrowly defined range of issues and regulations may have difficulty adjusting to these new requirements and responsibilities.

Extensive retraining may be required for some staff. In-service training to help staff accept new roles should focus first on changing attitudes and motivation and secondly on building necessarily skills (Melaville & Blank, 1991, citing the Annie E. Casey Foundation's *New Futures Initiative Strategic Planning Guide*). After staff have been allowed to express concerns and ask questions about proposed changes, they are likely to be more receptive to training in new policies and roles. Among the many skills needed for effective performance in these new roles will be knowledge of the service system, community organizing skills, clinical family skills and record-keeping, and administrative skills.

Differential pay scales may also be a source of staff dissention when agencies collaborate in projects by donating staff time to a single project. For instance, staff from government agencies and staff from non-profit agencies working together in a collaborative venture may have similar responsibilities but significantly different salaries and benefits. Conflict over this issue may be alleviated somewhat in the initial stages of a project by making staff participation voluntary and by stressing the innovative nature of the work. As projects grow and become more permanent, however, more equitable pay scales may be needed to preserve staff harmony.

Efforts to develop information-sharing systems and multi-program application and eligibility procedures must confront the complex confidentiality regulations and procedures. Yet in many cases, management operations, not actual confidentiality laws or regulations, are the major barriers to the exchange of confidential information (Hobbs, 1991). Furthermore, some legal barriers to sharing confidential information can be surpassed through *informed consent* documents. Release forms signed by clients may authorize certain types of information exchange (Joining Forces et al., 1992).

However, the issue of confidentiality is not simply one of rules and procedures. Melaville and Blank (1991) argue that, apart from crucial constitutional rights at stake, confidentiality is an important service issue since clients, especially those engaging in high-risk or illegal behavior, may not seek needed services if they feel that personal information will not be protected. Therefore, precautions should be taken beyond the legal requirements to assure that access to confidential information is limited to as small a number of staff as possible. To preserve trust, agencies may need to limit the exchange of information to only the most crucial elements and clients should have a clear sense of how information will be used, and by whom. Staff training should stress that failure to respect privileged information erodes trust between agencies and the communities they serve and that improper use of information could result in harm to clients.

INTERAGENCY SERVICE INTEGRATION

As noted earlier, the process of service integration can take place between agencies or within a single agency providing multiple services. In large umbrella agencies encompassing multiple programs, turf issues and competition between separate divisions may be as strong as those between separate agencies. Structural issues relating to service integration within umbrella agencies are discussed more fully in the next section.

Interagency efforts to integrate services generally fall under the label of collaboration (Bruner, 1991; Levy et al., 1992; Mattessich & Monsey, 1992). Bruner (1991) distinguishes interagency *collaboration* from commonly interchanged terms such as *communication* and *coordination*:

> *Communication* can help people do their jobs better by providing more complete information, but it does not require any joint activity. *Coordination* involves joint activity, but it allows individuals to maintain their own sets of goals, expectations, and responsibilities. In contrast, *collaboration requires the creation of joint goals to guide the collaborators' actions*. (p. 6)

In some cases, communication and coordination may be more appropriate strategies for interaction between agencies, especially when the agencies do not have a successful track record of collaborative efforts to build on. Discussion groups and coordinating councils can set the stage for future collaborative efforts. Focusing on state-level collaborative strategies, Bruner outlines three levels of interagency collaboration, which he terms first, second, and third generation approaches. These stages are outlined below:

> *First Generation Approaches.* Through the establishment of interagency groups (task forces, commissions, committees, or councils), state policy makers direct agencies to plan together to address child and family needs.

> *Second Generation Approaches.* States finance and provide guidance and technical assistance to local collaborative initiatives through multi-site demonstration projects. Sites are selected for their ability to develop models to meet child and family needs that could apply to other parts of the state.
>
> *Third Generation Approaches.* Building on experiences of multi-site demonstration projects, state policy makers design comprehensive, statewide collaborative approaches to meet child and family needs, incorporating strategies to develop the leadership base needed to support successful programs. States that have moved the farthest in developing statewide strategies for supporting local collaboration have recognized the need for new structures to nurture collaborative efforts and to develop methods for holding collaborative groups accountable for producing positive community outcomes. (p. 22)

First generation collaborative approaches are common throughout the human services. Agranoff (1991) notes that private agency community planning councils are being replaced in many localities by units anchored in local general-purpose governments. In some instances, interagency planning coalitions fostered through the service integration efforts of the 1970s have continued to function to the present. Coalitions function with various levels of formality and authority. Some have broad missions such as the development of goals and objectives for children and families, while others are structured around specific social issues such as homelessness or child injury prevention. In a study of nine such planning councils, Agranoff (1991) found that these groups were involved in a variety of service integration-related activities such as the development of services continuum for target populations, promoting new services in response to community crises, promoting the unification of selected services, and orchestrating community responses to various social crises.

Second generation collaborative approaches (multi-site pilot projects) have become increasingly common in many states. A notable example of second generation approaches is the proliferation of school-linked services projects. A convergence of forces has led to a wave of school-linked pilot projects that are transforming both the educational process and the way services are delivered to children and families (Kirst, 1992; Behrman, 1992; Kahn & Kamerman, 1992). Kahn and Kamerman (1992) summarize the major motivations behind the movement toward school-linked services as the need for *school readiness* and agency access to a *universal institution.* Overcoming a traditional tendency to consider students' social and health issues as peripheral to the educational process, many educators have become increasingly concerned about "school readiness," meaning that children cannot learn if they are not healthy and well-nourished or do not have stable family and community support networks (Bruner & Carter, 1991; Melaville, Blank, & Asayesh, 1993). While many schools have had counselors and school social workers in the past, some of these staff people have been cut in the midst of tight budgets, and those who remain are often overwhelmed by the complexity of student issues (i.e., gang violence, teen pregnancy, drug-exposed children, AIDS, child abuse cases, and mandates to provide individualized education plans for handicapped and severely emotionally disturbed students). The complexity of students' needs–and school districts' limited funds and expertise to address these needs–have made many educators increasingly receptive to on-site services by outside agencies.

At the same time, social and health agencies have become interested in schools because they are "universal" institutions, meaning that all children are required to attend school. The ability to provide services at the school site not only allows agencies access to the bulk of young people in a community, it also provides a relatively easy access point for other family members. It should be noted, however, that the concept of schools as a universal institution is most accurate when describing elementary and middle schools. By the time students reach high school, many of those with the most serious needs have dropped out.

While many school-based service projects focus primarily on a single issue area (dropout prevention, teen pregnancy, health education), an increasing number of operational multi-service centers have been established. Most of these centers seek to foster increased parent and community involvement in children's education and generally promote preventative interventions over traditional crisis-oriented approaches. The tradition of strong county governments makes local level demonstration projects (second generation approaches) a natural strategy in California.

San Diego's New Beginnings–a model for other projects throughout the state and country–provides a variety of family services, including some traditionally provided through school administration (i.e., eligibility determination for free and reduced price lunches), in a center staffed by city and county departments (New Beginnings Feasibility Study, 1990). Parents enroll children in the Hamilton School through the center, which conducts a family needs assessment for every child entering the school. Staff from participating county agencies are renamed *family service advocates*, and provide general assistance to families and help families obtain services not provided through the center. The New Beginnings model and other school-linked models are now being replicated throughout the state through a series of SB620 Healthy Start planning and demonstration project grants.

California's size, and the vast differences in the size and demographic composition of county populations, make statewide integration strategies difficult. Moving from series of pilot projects to a statewide integrated service network–Bruner's *Third Generation Approach*–requires a positive and cooperative relationship between state and local governments. In a time of state-wide fiscal crisis, the relationship between state and county governments in California has been seriously eroded. Many county governments, having been given new responsibilities with diminished resources to meet them, have developed internal service integration strategies to manage limited resources, but have become increasingly adversarial with state government.

Any moves toward statewide integrated service strategies will require a reexamination of the relationship between county, state, and federal government agencies. Creative fiscal strategies will be required to support programmatic reform (Center for the Study of Social Policy, 1991). For instance, more flexible funding and regulatory mechanisms need to be explored to allow counties to respond to local needs and utilize community-based preventative strategies. In 1989, the state moved in this direction with the passage of SB 997, which allowed counties which had developed interagency children's councils and adopted 3-year plans for coordinating children's services to request waivers of regulations which inhibit coordination (Chang et al., 1991). However, the implementing agencies at the state level were slow to establish a clear method for processing such waiver requests.

Some counties have begun to push for more radical shifts in financing approaches, requesting capitated billing rates for social and health service programs with increased county discretion on how funds are spent. New models based on managed health care have been proposed for social services. Some models, still in conception phases, have proposed the provision of services under a single organization, similar to a health maintenance organization with a broader scope of services. These emerging approaches have the potential to reconfigure the relationship between agencies and the communities and populations they serve, but future efforts toward a capitated billing system will require safeguards for clients.

SERVICE INTEGRATION WITHIN UMBRELLA AGENCIES

While service integration has been described primarily at the service delivery level, it is also important to assess service integration at the organizational level. In recent years, there has been a growing interest at the city and county level of local government in restructuring human service programs under one "umbrella" organization. However, to understand the origins of these ideas, it is necessary to highlight the experiences of state governments seeking to integrate human services under "umbrella" state agencies.

In the 1970s and early 1980s, state governments throughout the United States experimented with many different human service agency structures in an effort to create organizations that were more comprehensive, efficient, accessible, and consistent. The major thrust of most efforts was the creation of "umbrella agencies," or "superagencies," in which social services and other human services programs operated under one administrative structure. Among programs most commonly included under umbrella structures along with social services were public health, mental health, mental retardation, adult connections, youth institutions, vocational rehabilitation, and employment services (Chi, 1987).

By 1987, twenty-six states had established comprehensive human service agencies. The character of reorganization differed significantly from state to state, depending on the population, political framework and traditions of each area. The structure of these comprehensive agencies varied according to: (1) the level of comprehensiveness (number of programs provided under one administrative structure, (2) the degree of centralization (lines of authority and the relative autonomy of regional offices or county agencies), and (3) the degree of specialization vs. generalization (the extent to which the organizational structure emphasized special population issues vs. geographical or other general population criteria in the administration and delivery of services). A common trend in many states, however, was to consolidate program administration in some manner and to move toward a regionalized program with increasing power for generalist administrators overseeing a variety of programs.

As Chi (1987) notes, there is no one successful model for consolidating services since there are various strengths and limitations in different models adopted by the states. Chi developed the following typology to characterize the different structures of state human services agencies:

1. *Integrated central agency* which provides all or most administrative program authority of previously autonomous programs in a highly centralized structure.
2. *Consolidated central agency* organized along traditional program lines with an administrative unit which assists the agency head in establishing policy and goals.

3. *Confederated central agency* includes coordinated units which retain most autonomy and administrative authority.
4. *Noncomprehensive agency* in which social services such as income maintenance are administered separately from other human services with no central administrative or coordinating structure. (p. 26)

The first three agency types in Chi's typology can be considered umbrella or "comprehensive" agencies. According to Chi, of the twenty-five states that had some form of comprehensive umbrella agency in 1987, eight could be classified as integrated agencies (Alaska, Arizona, Arkansas, Delaware, Florida, Iowa, Kansas and North Dakota), thirteen maintained consolidated agencies (California, Georgia, Idaho, Kentucky, Louisiana, North Carolina, Oklahoma, Pennsylvania, Tennessee, Vermont, Virginia, Washington, and Wisconsin), and five had confederated agencies (Hawaii, Massachusetts, Nevada, Oregon, and Wyoming).

Since reorganizing large bureaucratic departments requires a good match between the expectations of politicians and the views of professionals about the needs of the community to be served, it is important to identify the criteria by which the success or failure of the restructured agency can be judged. Different program structures have strengths and limitations, and there are at least nine performance indicators for umbrella human service agencies (Ezell & Patti, 1990):

- *responsiveness to program constituencies* (ability to address the specific interests and needs of special population groups such as the developmentally disabled, children, the chronically mentally ill, frail elderly, etc.);
- *responsiveness to local political preferences* (sensitivity of agency to local traditions, political ideologies, and political leadership);
- *responsiveness to local needs* (ability of the agency to configure its services to the particular social problems and client populations found in an area);
- *equity in service provision and resource distribution* (availability of essential services for all who need them regardless of where they live);
- *client accessibility to multiple programs* (extent of collocation, speed and efficiency of client applications, multiple-program eligibility determination);
- *coordination and integration of services to clients* (integrated case management, ability to meet the complex and interconnected needs of 'multi-problem' families);

- *accountability to a central authority* (ability of central authority to monitor, evaluate, and control policy and resources);
- *maximizing efficiency* (the achievement of economies of scale, avoidance of duplication and elimination of administrative inefficiency); and
- *intra-interdepartment coordination* (facilitation of joint planning and interdepartmental program initiatives). (pp. 38-43)

While traditional specialized program structures may allow providers to tailor services toward the specific set of needs, a common criticism of these categorical programs is that they are too narrowly focused and fail to meet the needs of clients with multiple problems or issues. More centralized or consolidated administrative structures may increase comprehensiveness of services under one structure, but to provide services in a seamless fashion, it is necessary to integrate at the local level as well. Highly decentralized multi-service agencies, particularly those with single intake systems and collocated services, can help facilitate access to services for clients with multiple needs. For individuals and families seeking only a single service, however, the system may actually be more difficult to access. For instance if all potential clients seeking services from a multi-service center are required to undergo a comprehensive needs assessment, fill out lengthy forms, and be assigned to a case manager, individuals seeking only minimal services may need to spend far more time than they would otherwise and may or may not use the services. Therefore, integrated systems need to account for different levels of client needs and preferences in their intake procedures.

In addition, state human service agencies are sometimes criticized for failing to respond to local preferences, thereby failing to engender local ownership and involvement in services (Ezell & Patti, 1990). In contrast, community-based multi-service agencies, especially those that involve local "general purpose" governments in the planning and provision of services, are generally seen as responsive to local political preferences. Similarly, decentralized program structures are seen as responsive to local preferences and needs (e.g., social problems affecting client populations).

Although Ezell and Patti developed their nine performance indicators focusing on state-level umbrella agencies, these indicators may also be applied to county-level human agencies services. In California, with its large population and relatively autonomous county governments, the structure of county human service agencies, which actually deliver most services, varies significantly from county to county. Some county systems remain highly categorical, with several distinct human services agencies, while others are more comprehensive and consolidated. As with Chi's typology of state human service systems, county superagencies vary according to comprehensiveness, degree of centralization and degree of specialization.

Service integration lessons learned from state-level reorganizations can be applied selectively at the county level. Different government structures make the balance of power and the process of decision-making quite different at the county level. For instance, a central lesson from the state reorganizations was the gubernatorial involvement was essential to successful organizational consolidation. In county governments–with a non-elected professional administrator–the power dynamic is likely to be much different. The creation of a new superagency with a single director may be perceived as a loss of power for the county executive, who is unlikely to have sole authority to appoint the agency director. In a county system where a large proportion of governmental activity is focused on the delivery of services, the needs of a large human service superagency may prove to be a dominant force in county government.

Resistance to reorganization cannot be characterized simply as a power issue, however. While advocacy groups for special population groups may not be as large or well organized at the county level as they are at state and federal levels, professionals in specialized areas may see it as their responsibility to protect services for special populations. As a result, they may actively resist some types of county agency reorganization. Even when consolidation will not result in a loss of services, specialists may fear the loss of autonomy and control over service models. For instance, in a system that consolidates hospital services with public health, mental health and substance abuse services, professionals outside the hospital system may fear the imposition of medical models on services for population groups requiring complex social supports. In systems consolidating public health services with welfare–or income maintenance–services, public health professionals may fear the imposition of new models which emphasize eligibility for services over prevention (Nolan, 1989).

Cultivating support, and involvement from elected officials such as boards of supervisors, city leaders, and local elected boards–and educating them about the complexities of the service system–is essential to a smooth and sustaining reorganization. This idea was not always recognized by those involved in organizational reform at the state level. According to Lynn (1980), reformers "are apt to view politicians as sleeping lions who are not to be awakened if life and limb are to be preserved" (p. 73). Such a view is shortsighted, however, especially since organizational consolidation can significantly alter the balance of power within the county system. Making elected officials aware of the potential ramifications of change may help create a public forum for prioritizing organizational issues.

In county governments–as in state systems–the creation of efficient, accessible and effective superagency structures requires a mixture of political pragmatism, technical expertise, and long-term vision. While the ultimate structure of a superagency–with clear lines of authority and consistent administrative procedures–is important, the process for developing and operating such a system is equally important. Even the most well conceived service models will fail if strategy implementation issues are ignored. Figure 1 includes some of the strategic questions that may be of use at various stages in the creation and management of consolidated superagencies.

One reason that successful integration of services is often elusive is that reformers fail to set clear boundaries for their efforts. A criticism of the service integration efforts of the 1960s and 1970s was that these federally-initiated efforts, while based on a grandiose vision of a fully integrated service system, failed to set practical interim goals and account for the political realities of local areas. Service integration efforts that originated in the 1980s and 1990s–in what could be called a "second wave" of service integration–were generally initiated at local levels in response to practical needs. The various pilot projects have gradually grown into something of a national "movement." The fact that this movement emerged primarily from local sources is both a strength and a potential weakness.

The strength of the movement's grassroots origins is that it may be more sustainable than earlier "top-down" efforts, which virtually disappeared when national political leadership changed and attention shifted to other issues. While many current service integration projects will probably fall by the wayside, the diversity of projects hopefully will lead to some successful models that can be replicated. Efforts at replicating some "successful" projects–such as San Diego's New Beginnings and other school-linked service models–are already underway throughout California and the rest of the country.

A weakness in the current service integration movement, however, is that with so many competing local integration efforts, the movement itself is somewhat fragmented and may do little to remedy fragmentation at state and national levels. While service integration efforts need not–and indeed *should not*–be orchestrated entirely from the top down, it is essential that state and federal governments play an active supportive role, both in exploring new funding approaches and in helping coordinate efforts and facilitate communication to lessen fragmentation throughout the health and human services system. In a human service system covering a vast geographical and political landscape, attempts to integrate the entire range

FIGURE 1. Strategies for Organizing Human Service Agencies

I. MANAGING CHANGE FOR SERVICE INTEGRATION

A. *Why is reorganization needed?*

What is the impetus for reorganization (financial crisis, potential crisis, inefficiency, poor client outcomes, a vision for a better system)?

Is the rationale for reorganization realistic, persuasive, and commonly understood? How can this rationale be communicated to various constituencies?

B. *How much change is needed and when should changes occur?*

Should full-scale reorganization be pursued immediately, or is a more incremental strategy most appropriate?

What changes are required to alleviate crises? What changes will provide the most long-term benefits?

C. *Who must be involved in the change process?*

Who are the constituents of various categorical programs and what is their stake in the current system?

Are elected political leaders informed and involved in the process?

Who are the potential constituents of change and of a consolidated system?

II. DESIGNING INTEGRATIVE SUPERAGENCY STRUCTURES

A. *What are the strengths of the current system and how can they be preserved?*

How can the needs of existing program constituencies–especially those of the smallest, least powerful, or most stigmatized groups–be met under a consolidated system?

What protections can be assured for vulnerable population groups in a system that may be sensitive to volatile political forces?

B. *What are the limitations of the current system and how can they be eliminated?*

What are the areas of service duplication and how can services be more efficient?

Who is not being served adequately and how might their needs be met under a new system?

FIGURE 1 (continued)

How accessible are current services? Are services available to all who need them regardless of where they live? If not, how can services be restructured to improve access and equity of service provision?

Do agencies with similar client populations or interconnected service issues currently work together in a coordinated or integrated manner?

C. To whom should the agency be accountable?

What are the appropriate lines of authority within a superagency? Should the agency emphasize generalist or specialist administration?

What are the appropriate lines of authority within the county system? To whom will the superagency director be accountable? How will the superagency structure affect the balance of power within the county?

How can tensions between local political preferences and professional assessment of local needs be resolved?

How can a consolidated agency meet fragmented reporting and regulatory requirements of state and federal programs? In what areas can and should waivers be sought?

How is the superagency likely to be perceived in local neighborhoods and communities?

of services at once are destined to fail. Even when focusing on a distinct and manageable geographic area, service integration efforts need to begin with a strategic focus on a particular set of issues or services. As Kahn and Kamerman (1992) note, "Except in quite small towns, it is simply not feasible to organize all major and minor institutions affecting families and children into one overall, complete delivery system . . . even in small towns this may not necessarily be desirable" (p. 35). They suggest a deliberate focus on clusters of issues with the most potential to benefit from service integration. As a starting point for further discussion, they offer the following possibilities for cluster areas:

- *Cluster #1: Programs offering access to money and resources on a means-tested basis.* This cluster includes Medicaid, AFDC, general assistance, food stamps, low-income energy assistance, WIC, special housing assistance, and emergency shelters and housing. Reconciling inconsistent eligibility rules would facilitate integrated service mechanisms such as single application forms and procedures, staff co-location and easier sharing of staff.

- *Cluster #2: Services for adolescents.* This cluster includes education about teen pregnancy and parenting, substance abuse prevention and treatment, delinquency prevention and treatment, mental health treatment, alternative schools, drop-out prevention, and vocational training. Natural linkages exist in many of these issue areas and different programs frequently serve the same clients.
- *Cluster #3: Services for children under age 12.* This cluster includes efforts to integrate services within the child welfare system, such as protective services, foster care, family preservation, counseling, respite care and parent education. Also, this cluster would encompass efforts to link services across categorical systems, such as child welfare, mental health, special education, and juvenile justice. While the ideal situation is to have services integrated *within* systems before attempting *cross-system* linkages, it may be more realistic to begin some cross-system linkages in highly related areas while attempting to integrate within systems. (Kahn & Kamerman, 1992, p. 36, paraphrased.)

These cluster areas can serve as a "jumping-off" point for strategic thinking about services that might realistically be linked within a local or regional service system. Yet even selection of a clearly-defined range of issues or programs for initial integration efforts is not enough. Planning for "nuts and bolts" issues (e.g., administrative structures, confidentiality agreements, differential pay scales, and training staff for new roles) is necessary to make collaborative models successful.

CONCLUSION

As should be clear from the preceding discussion, service integration cannot be defined by a particular service model or outcome, but instead should be conceived of as an ongoing reform process seeking to make the human service system more effective in meeting the needs of families and communities. Experience shows that service integration is unlikely to produce significant financial savings in the short term because of the investment in time and effort required to successfully integrate policy, staff, and financial processes. Attempts to use services integration as a tool to alleviate short-term financial crises are likely to result in failure. However, well-designed and implemented efforts with a long-term vision and realistic interim goals may be able to produce significant dividends in the form of reduced duplication and waste, strengthened local communities, and improved client outcomes through prevention and more effective interventions. A thorough understanding of the evolution of service integration issues can provide a significant foundation for envisioning a totally restructured neighborhood-based and city/county human service system for the future.

REFERENCES

Agranoff, R. (1991, November/December). Human services integration: Past and present challenges in public administration. *Public Administration Review, 51* (No. 6).

Agranoff, R., & Pattakos, A.N. (1979). *Dimensions of services integration*. Rockville, MD: Project SHARE Monographs.

American Society for Public Administration. (1974). *Human services integration*. Washington, DC: ASPA Special Project Report.

Behrman, R. (Ed.). (1992, Spring). School-linked services. *The future of children*. Center for the Future of Children. *2*(1).

Bruner, C. (1991). *Thinking collaboratively: Ten questions and answers to help policy makers improve children's services*. Washington, DC: Education and Human Services Consortium.

Bruner, C., & Carter, J. (1991). *Family support and education: A holistic approach to school readiness*. National Conference of State Legislators.

Center for the Study of Social Policy. (1991). *Leveraging dollars, leveraging change: Refinancing and restructuring children's services in five sites*. Washington, DC: CSSP.

Chang, H.N. et al. (1991). *Fighting fragmentation: Collaborative efforts to serve children and families in California's counties*. San Francisco: California Tomorrow and the Children and Youth Policy Project.

Chi, K. (1987). What has happened to the comprehensive human services agency? *New England Journal of Human Services*, *8*(3), 24-31.

Council of State Governments. (1974). *Human services integration: State functions in implementation*. Lexington, KY: CSG.

Ezell, M., & Patti, R.J. (1990). State human service agencies: Structure and organization. *Social Service Review, 64*(1), 22-45.

The Family Impact Seminar (FIS). (1991). *Coordination, collaboration, integration: Strategies for serving families more effectively*. Washington, DC: FIS.

Gardner, S. (1976). *Roles for general purpose governments in services integration*. Rockville, MD: Project SHARE Monographs.

Hobbs, L.J. (1991). *Tackling the confidentiality barrier: A practical guide for integrated family services*. Department of Social Services, County of San Diego, Community Relations Bureau.

Horton, G.T., Carr, V.M.E., & Corcoran, G.J. (1976). *Illustrating services integration from categorical bases*. Rockville, MD: Project SHARE Monographs.

John, D. (1977). *Managing the human services system: What have we learned from services integration*. Rockville, MD: Project SHARE Monographs.

Joining Forces et al. (1992). *Confidentiality and collaboration: Information sharing in interagency efforts.* Denver: Education Commission of the States Distribution Center.

Kahn, A.J., & Kamerman, S.B. (1992). *Integrating services integration: An overview of initiatives, issues, and possibilities.* New York: National Center for Children in Poverty.

Kirst, M.W. (1992). *Changing the system for children's services: Building linkages with schools.* Washington, DC: Council of Chief State School Officers.

Kusserow, R.P. (1991). *Services Integration: A Twenty Year Retrospective.* Washington, DC: U.S. Department of Health and Human Services, Office of the Inspector General.

Kusserow, R.P. (1992). *Services integration for families and children in crisis.* Washington, DC: U.S. Department of Health and Human Services, Office of the Inspector General.

Levy, J.E., Kagan, S.L., & Copple, C. (1992). *Are we ready? Collaboration to support young children and their families.* Washington, DC: Joining Forces.

Lynn, L.E. Jr. (1980). *The state and human services: Organizational change in a political context.* Cambridge, MA: The Massachusetts Institute of Technology.

Mattessich, P., & Monsey, B. (1992). *Collaboration: What makes it work–A review of research literature on factors influencing successful collaboration.* Amherst H. Wilder Foundation.

Melaville, A., & Blank, M. (1991). *What it takes: Structuring interagency partnerships to connect children and families with comprehensive services.* Washington, DC: Education and Human Services Consortium.

Melaville, A., Blank, M., & Asayesh, G. (1993). *Together we can: A guide for crafting a profamily system of education and human services.* U.S. Department of Education and U.S. Department of Health and Human Services.

National Academy of Public Administration. (1977). *Reorganization in Florida: How is services integration working*? Report by a Panel of the National Academy of Public Administration.

Nolan, P.A. (1989). Primary prevention with the poor: Structural conflicts between the health and welfare systems. *Journal of Health & Social Policy, 1*(1), 99-103.

San Diego Department of Social Services. (1990). *New Beginnings Feasibility Study.* San Diego, CA: Department of Social Services.

Soler, M., & Shauffer, C. (1990). Fighting fragmentation: Coordination of services for children and families. *University of Nebraska Law Review, 69*(2).

United States General Accounting Office. (1992). *Integrating human services: Linking at-risk families with services more successful and system reform efforts.* Gaithersburg, MD: U.S.G.A.O.

Marking Progress Toward Service Integration: Learning to Use Evaluation to Overcome Barriers

John O'Looney, PhD

SUMMARY. While federal statutes defining categorical programs and funding streams are most often cited as barriers to service integration efforts, there is evidence that service integration efforts are also being stymied by factors at the state and local levels as well. This case study examines five types of barriers to service integration that have been evident in Georgia's Family Connection and describes how an evaluation instrument and process was developed to assess progress toward service integration at the local level. The findings of a pilot study of the use of this instrument suggest that it can help to: (a) define starting points for service integration efforts; (b) identify specific service integration activities that are feasible in the context of a unique community; (c) specify the time needed to be allocated to service integration efforts; (d) identify the local costs and benefits of engaging in service integration; and (e) provide specifications for conducting a self-assessment of progress at the local

John O'Looney is Human Services Research Associate, Carl Vinson Institute of Government, The University of Georgia, 201 North Milledge Avenue, Athens, GA 30602.

Materials for the case study used in this research were drawn from the evaluation of the State of Georgia's Family Connection Initiative. Dr. O'Looney is the program evaluator for the initiative.

[Haworth co-indexing entry note]: "Marking Progress Toward Service Integration: Learning to Use Evaluation to Overcome Barriers." O'Looney, John. Co-published simultaneously in *Administration in Social Work* (The Haworth Press, Inc.) Vol. 21, No. 3/4, 1997, pp. 31-65; and: *Human Services Integration* (ed: Michael J. Austin) The Haworth Press, Inc., 1997, pp. 31-65. Single or multiple copies of this article are available for a fee from The Haworth Document Delivery Service [1-800-342-9678, 9:00 a.m. - 5:00 p.m. (EST). E-mail address: getinfo@haworth.com].

level toward service integration goals. *[Article copies available for a fee from The Haworth Document Delivery Service: 1-800-342-9678. E-mail address: getinfo@haworth.com]*

INTRODUCTION

Service integration represents a veritable "holy grail" for many in the human services professions. Unfortunately, besides the existence of promising models of re-engineering in the business world, there are few or no effective economic or social forces promoting service integration. Unlike corporations that are free to contract with, merge with, or buy outright other businesses in order to rationalize operations, service agencies are generally constrained by law and narrowly defined funding streams from transforming the organizational environment (O'Looney, 1993b).[1] Moreover, while corporations are propelled by the profit motive to refine their operations, there is no comparable mechanism in the human services world that would compel trans-agency re-engineering. Calls for service agencies being jointly accountable for the welfare of *whole* families, rather than individually accountable for a single category of individual well-being, represent an attempt to provide such a motive for system change (Friedman, 1995). Even without strong structural incentives, human service managers are often motivated to act in concert. In recent years, such confederational activity has been referred to most often under the rubrics of "collaboration" and "services integration." Although in common usage there is considerable overlap in these terms, analytically speaking, collaboration refers to partnership formation that is believed to bring about change, while service integration (SI) refers to specific changes believed to make the system more efficient, effective, and comprehensive.

This case study uses the experience of a statewide human services initiative, Georgia's Family Connection (FC), to explore the dynamics of the relationship between collaboration and service integration. In particular, five potential explanations for the seeming failure of collaboration to lead to substantial integration of services are posited. The role of these five explanations is examined in terms of the development and piloting of an instrument for evaluating progress toward SI. Some tentative conclusions regarding the use of evaluation tools to support the movement toward service integration are drawn.

From Collaboration to Service Integration: In the best of worlds, collaboration grows out of a system of positive interdependence, in which the success of one agency's services for families fosters success at another agency which feeds back to the first agency, and so on (Tjosvold, 1986).

However, interagency collaboration can also be maintained for reasons that are relatively unrelated to family well-being, e.g., because it provides a means of political support (Gray, 1989), or a larger arena for power than exists in a single agency; or because it is naturally generated through daily interactions (Ellickson, 1991). With no structural mechanism driving non-profit collaboration, SI in human service environments may depend on chance dynamics, public sector entrepreneurism, and windows of opportunity (Kingdon, 1984). Perhaps because collaboration is so much more context dependent in the human services arena than in the for-profit sector, the literature on collaboration (and its cognates of interorganizational activity, partnerships, confederations, etc.) is so much richer and diverse.

Doubts About Value of Collaboration: Despite our deepening understanding of collaborative processes (Gray, 1985; Tjosvold, 1986; O'Looney, 1994a), there is still considerable doubt among agency administrators as to whether collaboration will in fact lead to re-engineered service delivery systems. There are two basic sources of this doubt: first, is the belief that the rewards of collaboration may not exceed the value of the time, effort, and resources expended on maintaining the communication links, organizational structure and administrative overhead of the collaborative; second, is the suspicion that many of the functions performed by collaboratives may have only tangential effects on the lives of troubled families. That is, collaboratives often act as additional layers of rule-making and paperwork, an escape from the agency-specific restrictions on programs and narrowly-defined professional roles, advocates for human services in general, and arenas that sustain substantial amounts of interpersonal conflict and drama. While one of these attendant attributes of collaboratives–helping professionals to be more flexible–has been shown to benefit service consumers (Schorr, 1989), the value of other attendant features of collaboration is less well established. It should be recognized that these attendant features are part of the package of moving from loosely structured "interagency cooperation" to a more tightly organized collaboration, which demands that agency resources become subject to joint strategic assessment, pooling, and program planning (Bruner, 1991). However, just like interagency cooperation before it, service collaboratives have disappointed many in the field because initial expectations have not been fulfilled (Gardner, 1995). Some of this disappointment has occurred because collaboration has been incompletely realized. Though able to develop broad mission statements with some ease, and with effort, to develop and manage new programs with new resources, substantial sharing of existing resources and strategic evaluation and redirection of existing programs have been rare even in the better collaboratives (O'Looney, 1992).

In assessing the lack of progress toward service integration, it is necessary to understand that in addition to the difficulty agencies have collaborating, categorical funding streams make *comprehensive* service integration a near impossibility. Nevertheless, even assuming that under current law only 10-20% of agency budgets can be redirected so as to support a more integrated service system, the record of effective redeployment of these resources is still poor. Only rarely have collaboratives taken the first studying and planning steps toward SI, e.g., using tools such as "client data matches," which reveal the extent to which different agencies serve the same clients or seriously analyze service overlaps that are ripe for re-engineering (Gardner, 1995). Fewer still have taken steps to reconfigure direct service workers' job duties, work flows, and authority in response to such studies (Kraus & Pillsbury, 1993; O'Looney, 1993a; O'Looney, 1996).

In the near future, it is likely that the major structural barrier to SI presented by categorical federal funding streams may be removed. If this occurs, state and local human service collaboratives will still face a number of more psychological obstacles. As Senge (1990) has pointed out, however, reworking "mental models" can often be as or more important to learning organizations than removing structural obstacles. Drawing on years of participant observation in service collaboration efforts, I have identified five such mental model barriers.

These five "explanations for failure" are presented in the order of "most benign" to "least benign." Explanations that are "benign" are ones that do not imply fault or any active efforts on the part of collaborative partners to block system-change. This ordering is important because benign explanations suggest that fairly simple, gentle and non-directive efforts on the part of state-level SI entrepreneurs can be effective. Benign explanations imply that by simply setting the right tone and focus, state leaders can support the emergence of SI from the bottom-up. In contrast, less benign explanations will generally demand a more top-down, directive role on the part of state leaders.

Five Explanations for the Failure of Collaboration to Lead to Service Integration

1) Lack of Time: The most benign explanation is that collaborative partners simply run out of time to deal with SI strategies such as redeploying staff, sharing training and other resources, or developing cross-agency client tracking systems. After partners share basic program information, establish and nurture collaborative governance structures, and develop and manage joint grant programs, there is little time left to study and take action on redeployment possibilities. Gardner (1992) has called this syndrome *projectitis* or the tendency to be so caught up in the details of implementing specific projects that the larger reconfiguration and SI goals are never undertaken.

2) Lack of Clear Definitions and Identifiable Starting Points: It is possible that, to the average human service manager, the concepts of service integration, redeployment, and re-engineering are essentially abstractions. As such, these managers may have trouble identifying concrete activities that represent a starting point for the realization of the SI goal. Service integration efforts die for lack of such a starting point. Moreover, when SI concepts are abstract, different individuals will fill in the "black box" with different particular meanings. For some, SI will mean working together on a jointly designed program, for others it will mean developing a common client information system. With these different mental models in action, it becomes nearly impossible to get meaningful answers to the question, "Are services integrated in your community?"

3) Lack of State and Local Leadership: The literature on SI emphasizes the importance of leaders learning from past mistakes (Kagan, 1993), building commitment to the process, and overcoming technical barriers (Jennings & Krane, 1994; Jennings, 1994). The lack of leadership presents a somewhat less benign explanation for SI failure in that one assumes that state human service executives can communicate to local collaborative partners that SI is a high priority. Similarly, when SI efforts fail because local human service leaders have not requested permission for, help with, or clarification of specific SI mechanisms, their inactivity is in some degree a matter of choice. As the Family Connection went through the Pew Charitable Trusts' Children's Initiative process, the importance of state-local collaboration and joint leadership for system change was highlighted. As will become clear in the case study that follows, joint leadership for system change is inherently difficult to define and maintain. This is the case because leadership on the part of one group such as state level Family Connection partners implies a certain degree of "followship" on the part of local level members. Essentially, it is difficult for leadership to be exerted simultaneously from the top-down and from the bottom-up. However, the literature on implementation suggests that strategies that allow for some balance between these two directions of leadership may be more effective than strategies that exclusively emphasize one direction (Sabatier, 1986).

4) Lack of a Positive Benefit-Cost Ratio: A still less benign explanation is that partners in collaborative organizations essentially do not believe that redeployment is either possible or, if possible, worth the effort. On one hand, this explanation is based on the idea that there are a number of practical and policy barriers to redeployment that cannot easily be overcome; categorical funding streams, confidentiality guidelines, sunk costs in existing training and technologies, and the inability to change system-wide personnel policies are frequently mentioned in this regard. On the other hand, even if such barriers could be overcome, there are some who question whether the cost of overcoming the barriers will be worth the benefits. Both the barrier-scaling and cost-benefit questions represent potentially testable hypotheses. In order to conduct such cost-benefit tests, however, two pieces of developmental work will need to be done. First, we will need to know what resources are truly redeployable and what resources can only be used as they are currently deployed. If we discover, for example, that only 3% of the combined agency and non-profit budgets for improving the lives of children and families can be redeployed, the potential return on redirection strategies is likely to be much less than if 20% or 30% of such budgets are potentially redeployable. Secondly, there is a need to define more exactly the benefit side of the cost-benefit equation. Currently, measures of benefits–the outcomes, impacts, or results of human service activity–are highly underdeveloped. Typically, an individual agency is able to provide client statistics (or process data) related to the program the agency operates. Even when impact data are available, there is usually not a standard against which to interpret the data. For example, we may know that a program improvement effort costing two million dollars was able to reduce teen pregnancy by 5% among an at-risk population of 15,000 youth, but what we do not know is whether this improvement is a bargain or a waste of resources. In order to know whether a program is a bargain or a waste, states and communities need to arrive at some consensus as to their "willingness to pay" for improved outcomes. Specifically, they must be able to assign a standardized value to particularly desirable results. The existence of "outcome prices" would provide human service managers with a benchmark against which to compare the cost of investing in SI efforts. For example, if the community and consumers value "one-stop" services (which save time and reduce hassles for consumers and insure more comprehensive treatment for families in need) at $5 per capita, this may or may not pay for implementing a one-stop service approach. It could, however, bring a certain concreteness and reality to discussions of the costs and benefits of service integration.

5) Threat to Security: The least benign explanation for the lack of SI activity is that collaborative partners fear that redeployment will undermine their power, status, and security. Power, status, and security rest on the organizational pillars of job descriptions, defined expertise, office locations, established hierarchies, and specified compensation and benefits packages. SI redeployment could threaten all of these pillars, and in one of the few cases where substantial redeployment of mainline agency personnel was carried out, a number of the employees who were retrained and assigned new duties reacted negatively to the change. Essentially, when it was decided to create a unified and generic case management system out of a number of more categorical programs and case management functions in Northampton County, Pennsylvania, the resistance among the direct service personnel was such that the plan was abandoned after only months of operation. In particular, service workers complained about having to deal with new client populations, being moved to new locations, and being stripped of the status they had achieved through specialization (Human Organization Science Institute, 1990). The fact that SI was so difficult in Northampton County, where the power to integrate services was within the scope of a single agency's authority, should temper optimism among those who believe that collaboration can easily achieve SI goals. It is likely that many human services executives who are somewhat reluctant participants in collaboratives instinctively realize that attempts to change systems within a collaborative (rather than a single agency) context will be more difficult than the promoters of collaboration generally realize.

These five hypothesized explanations for human services collaboratives failing to make progress in integrating services are not mutually exclusive. Rather, it is likely that all five have some explanatory power, depending on the context and stage of collaborative development, as seen in this case study of the initial steps taken by one state to support local SI efforts. It includes an analysis of these steps in light of the hypothesized explanations for the lack of progress toward service integration, the relatively benign quality of the explanations, and the support strategies (bottom-up versus top-down) such explanations evoke from state SI leaders.

THE CASE

As Agranoff (1991) and Kagan (1993) outline, the SI movement has roots going back to the Economic Opportunity Act of 1964. For the most part, however, efforts to integrate services have rarely kept up with the growth in new categories of service and have only had on-again, off-again support at the federal level. During the latter part of the '80s and the early '90s, interest in SI revived.[2] These contemporary SI efforts are more modest in scope and scale than earlier efforts (Agranoff, 1991) but more realistic in their approach to linking program research with operations implementation and management. Within the contemporary SI movement, states are experimenting with a variety of implementation strategies. California and Kentucky have developed uniform statewide approaches. In Kentucky, for example, legislation outlines the development of a system of family centers in every community. Other states such as Georgia have been less directive. In Georgia, communities are given considerable leeway to identify service collaborative goals and to employ the strategies that they believe best fit their unique political, cultural, and economic environments. Collaboration is encouraged through the awarding of grants to communities who have gone through a collaborative planning process which includes efforts to identify some SI goals. However, there is no expectation that such SI goals take any particular form. The following case describes an attempt by the State of Georgia to facilitate a more systematic approach to helping communities to identify and pursue SI goals.

Since 1990, the State of Georgia has supported the Family Connection (FC) initiative, a human services collaborative for improving the lives of children and families. At the state level, the collaborative combines the efforts of the departments of Human Resources, Education, Medical Assistance and Children and Youth Services, and at the community level, combines the efforts of both these state service agencies and a broad range of other organizations and businesses interested in the welfare of families. The initiative was designed to promote early intervention, family-centered, and community-based services. At the state level, the work of the FC is spearheaded by a team of site facilitators, who assist local collaboratives with planning, a Finance Committee, and an Evaluation Committee. While all three groups have an interest in promoting service integration, this case study is focused on the efforts of the Evaluation Committee. Membership in this committee represented a diverse mix of program managers, collaboration facilitators, and university faculty. The work of the Evaluation Committee in promoting SI was constrained in a couple of important ways. First, because of the paucity of experience both nationally and at the state level with actual implementation of many of the SI mechanisms, Evaluation Committee members were essentially no more enlightened about the potential for and costs of SI than members of the local collaboratives, and in some respects, these committee members were less knowledgeable about the prospects for implementing SI in unique local settings. Acknowledging this ignorance, the Evaluation Committee took a number of steps to study collaboration and SI and to place the findings of its investigations in a digestible context. These efforts can be grouped into three phases.

I. Describe the working of the state and local collaboratives and develop a model of collaboration. (O'Looney, 1994)

II. Systematically survey Family Connection partners at both the state and local level regarding collaboration and service integration. At the end of this phase, the committee realized that accurately measuring SI achievements would demand a substantial investment in refining concepts and building instruments. (O'Looney, 1994)

III. Assist collaboratives in measuring progress toward their own program goals; and create a "toolbox" of evaluation instruments for measuring progress toward system change goals. This latter effort has centered on the development of "Markers of Progress Toward Service Integration," an instrument for assessing to what degree individual FC communities are moving toward an integrated service system.[3] The third phase of the evaluation coincided with a rapid expansion of the number of local FC sites. Because of this expansion, FC collaboratives no longer shared a similar developmental history. Instead, FC communities were sorted into original, new implementation, and planning sites.

Top-Down versus Bottom-Up Leadership: In addition to being constrained by ignorance of the meaning of collaboration and SI, the Evaluation Committee was also constrained by a lack of consensus or shared understanding as to the nature of its leadership role vis-à-vis the local collaboratives. Traditionally, state-level leadership in implementing human service programs was realized through various command-and-control structures, one of which was an evaluation design issued from the top down (Sabatier, 1986). Because Family Connection principles declared that the FC initiative was to be community-based, the committee members realized that a traditional approach to evaluation would not be appropriate. One consequence of this realization was an agreement negotiated early on between local and state-level evaluation representatives that the local collaboratives would be responsible for program impact measures, while the state would evaluate collaboration and SI. However, even within the area designated as its responsibility, state-level Evaluation Committee members wanted to approach the evaluation design in a more bottom-up rather than top-down fashion. The theme of trust building between the state and local partners was prominent in this regard, and the Evaluation Committee felt strongly that the state evaluation process should not interfere with or undermine this trust. An operational outcome of this theme was the maxim that state and local partners "build it together." At the same time, however, because the committee members over time had gained substantially in knowledge of collaboration and SI, and because phase two evaluation findings indicated a lack of substantial progress toward SI goals, they also felt a need to exert more leadership especially with respect to new sites.

Understanding the tension felt by Evaluation Committee members who believe in both a bottom-up philosophy of nurturing local leadership and the desire to exert more top-down state leadership is important to understanding how and why an Evaluation Committee task group went about developing and testing the Markers of Progress Toward Service Integration instrument. The remainder of this case study focuses on: (1) creation of the Markers instrument; (2) its potential purposes; (3) the assumptions on which the instrument is based; and (4) the results of a piloting of the instrument in four communities. Throughout the discussion, an attempt is made to understand the role of the five explanations (for the lack of progress toward SI) in the development and testing of the Markers instrument and to describe how the tension between the desire for both top-down and bottom-up leadership played itself out in this process. (Cognates for the five explanations are italicized in the text to notify the readers that one of these mental models is being referenced.)

THE MARKERS

Creation of the Markers: The results of the collaboration/SI survey in phases one and two of the evaluation indicated that few sites had pooled funding beyond the funding provided in the collaboration grant and that even fewer sites had taken any significant steps toward such SI ideals as "one-stop shopping." More particularly, impetus for creating the markers also came from increased exposure (e.g., through work with the National Center for Service Integration) to knowledge about the scope and complexity of service integration.

Such exposure suggested to the state-level leaders of the FC that a key barrier to SI was the *lack of clear definitions and identifiable starting points* for making progress toward service integration. After examining the literature on SI, the task group charged with developing the Markers agreed to use Agranoff's (1991) four levels of service integration–the direct service level, the program level, the policy level, and the organizational level–as a framework. Use of Agranoff's typology tended to have two effects: first, it helped to generate a more comprehensive catalog and more *clearly defined* categories of SI efforts than would otherwise have been the case. Second, as will be clarified below, Agranoff's typology helps to sort out types of SI efforts that would demand specialized attention by personnel acting at different levels of organizational control. Such sorting of service integration into areas of service, program, policy, and organizational responsibility provides a certain degree of tactical assistance in *identifying starting points* for SI efforts.

The survey of service integration conducted during the second phase of the FC evaluation indicated that the Likert scale used to rate achievement of each component was not adequately grounded in concrete events (O'Looney, 1994b). Without such grounding, different respondents could rate the same situation differently based on their individual expectations of what could realistically be achieved as a result of an SI effort. Hence, in creating the Markers of Progress toward Service Integration (hereafter, the Markers), it was considered important to develop a scale of measuring progress on each marker (or SI feature) that would be meaningfully grounded in events, rather than perceptions. The measurement scale that resulted allows community respondents to define progress in four areas: studying and gaining consensus, planning, developing integration pilot projects, and implementing a service integration feature or features in mainline agencies.

Although Figure 1 suggests that service integration would develop sequentially (from studying to prototyping to implementation in mainline agencies), there are cases where this sequence can be jump started due to an SI feature already existing in an agency. Because this agency has already conducted some prototyping of the idea, they may be able to mentor other agencies through the process. The sample scale provided in Figure 1 for assessing implementation is designed to identify progress at a fairly global level. As partnerships go through, for example, a 2-3 year prototyping process, it would make sense to have one or more sub-scales to measure progress during this period. Although not shown in Figure 1, the Markers' process also asks that communities identify the particular organizations that have implemented an SI marker and the date at which partial or full implementation is thought to occur. In this way, it will be possible to track progress in at a more detailed level.

Purposes: In deciding on the purposes of the Markers document, the task group was split into two basic camps. On one side were those who believed that the Markers provided an ideal way to begin to define some SI standards for becoming and remaining a Family Connection community. Persons holding this opinion generally believed that service integration and system change efforts, not specific programming, were the defining features of the Family Connection. The suggested use of the Markers to establish standards in this way could be compared to the way companies use trademark and franchise standards to maintain quality and a customer base. In this view, in order to continue to call oneself an FC community, it would be necessary at certain stages of development to have reached a specific set or number of SI goals.

In developing a rationale for using the Markers to protect the value of

FIGURE 1. Sample Scale of Response Categories for Assessing Implementation of Service Integration Markers

STUDYING AND GAINING CONSENSUS		PLANNING		IMPLEMENTATION IN SERVICE PROTOTYPE		IMPLEMENTATION IN MAINLINE AGENCIES				
identified the feasibility and priority of each SI Marker	*organized task forces—no planning yet*	*initial planning only*	*detailed planning, begin implementation in a year*	*partial implementation in prototype*	*fully implemented in prototype—not elsewhere*	*partial implementation in 2+ agencies*	*partial implementation in 50+ % of agencies*	*full implementation in 1-2 agencies*	*full implementation in 50% of agencies*	*Completely Implemented in all partner agencies*
Early Development				*Midterm Development*						*Full Development*

the FC trademark, the group proposing this idea relied on a combination of three of the five SI failure explanations discussed above: the *lack of clear definitions and starting points*, the *lack of time*, and the *lack of sufficient state leadership*. In essence, this group believed that one of the chief reasons for local sites experiencing a lack of time to conduct SI experiments was that the state level collaborative leaders had not made a concerted effort to define clear expectations of SI achievements. This belief was bolstered by earlier collaboration survey findings indicating that:

- local collaborative goals were often not ambitious or specific enough to lead to effective action;
- goals tended to be project-oriented, rather than system-change oriented;
- middle managers in mainline (state) human service agencies have not subscribed to the goals.

This standard-setting group felt that establishing clear and challenging SI standards for FC communities would more effectively support local collaboration coordinators' efforts to engage service agency middle managers. Simultaneously, such a signal that a certain level of SI achievement was expected would notify local agency executives that continued FC funding would be dependent on their supporting SI effort. The basic mental model of the group arguing for this point of view was that the lack of time to work on service integration was not the result of cynicism or skepticism among middle managers about the *cost-benefit ratio* or *threat to security* of SI efforts; rather, for the most part this group thought that lack of time was more the result of local agency heads and state agency middle managers being pulled in numerous directions by the latest grant opportunity, program idea, or day-to-day operational crisis.

However, there was a small "realist" subset of this standard-setting group that believed that the lack of follow through on SI was due to influences less benign than a simple lack of time. Relying on evidence from phase one evaluation interviews, this realist group pointed out that the reluctance of some managers to work actively on SI tasks was due to these managers being skeptical about the capability of the collaborative to achieve the desired results within reasonable costs. This skepticism was particularly evident among managers with regard to the ability of refinancing schemes to draw down substantial funds.

It is probably important to observe that none of the task group members expressed a concern that SI efforts were being held up because of a sense of threat to the security of existing personnel. It could be that no one raised this specter because front-line personnel in Georgia's human service system were generally viewed as flexible and open to change. Some of the early case study data supported this view. Front-line Department of Family and Children Services personnel in one community, for example, expressed envy of the more generalist Family Connection services coordinators who were permitted to work with entire families in a holistic manner. However, in comparison to FC services coordinator roles, the specialty work of staff from this department tends to be either of low status (e.g., intake and eligibility) or to be characterized by a high level of stress and burn out (e.g., child protective services).

Although at certain times during the development of the Markers, the task group agreed that the Markers *might* be used as an assessment tool for determining the level of future funding of community collaboratives, the majority of the task group did not believe that the Markers should, at least initially or in the near term, be used in this manner. Moreover, the task group did not include "assessment for funding purposes" in the final list of Marker purposes. Instead, the purpose of the Markers instrument was to be primarily, if not solely, self-assessment. The Markers would be a tool around which communities would plan, implement, and chart progress on SI efforts. In the long-term, the task group expressed the hope that as experience with the Markers deepened and as a substantial database of SI efforts was established, it might be possible for local collaboratives to model themselves after other communities. That is, communities could learn from other similarly situated communities who seemed to have achieved more in terms of particular service integration goals.

When we consider the mental models implied by the decision not to have the Markers function as either a standard-setting or resource allocation tool, it is clear the Markers' task group as a whole relied chiefly on the *lack of time* and *lack of definitions and identifiable starting points* explanations for the slow progress toward service integration. Implicitly, it was assumed that with time, good starting points and a willingness to self-assess, local collaboratives would develop the leadership needed and would not encounter significant resistance due to skepticism as to *benefit costs* or a sense of *threat to security or status*. Being based on the most benign of the SI failure explanations, the official statement of Marker purposes ultimately represented a belief in a bottom-up strategy for using the Markers to support SI efforts.

Assumptions: In distributing the Markers of Progress for community use, three assumptions about SI were outlined and published along with the markers. The first assumption was that movement toward effective service integration is likely to be unique in each community. As such it was noted that one yardstick is insufficient to gauge the scope and depth of collaborative activities in Georgia's communities. Conceptually, the task group imagined an electronic version of the Markers where numerous and customized sub-measures could be established for each SI marker. In this manner, communities could begin to build their own yardstick against which to measure their achievement. The key theory underlying this community uniqueness assumption is that in allowing communities to customize the instrument, local leadership will be more likely to own the results. As such, this feature of the Markers process relies heavily on the lack of local leadership explanation. By allowing for local flexibility, the task group decided that the Markers instrument should work from the bottom up to elicit local leadership.

A second assumption outlined in the Markers' document is that some amount of resources will be dedicated explicitly to service integration and "that communities entering into a collaborative initiative will make available (in-kind or otherwise) resources equivalent to or greater than the resources provided by the state." By including these statements about the need to address one's SI efforts with adequate resources, the Markers document touches on, but does not fully respond to the *cost-benefit* explanation for the lack of progress in moving toward SI. The implication of these statements is that communities wishing to make progress will be able to do so if they identify SI projects in which they can afford to invest. The Markers document, however, does not provide guidance on how to address the more difficult cost-benefit issue of whether the investment in particular SI efforts will provide an adequate return.

The third assumption outlined in the Markers document is that local collaborative partners are committed to creating and maintaining their SI experiments for a number of years *after* the glue monies have ceased. This assumption is based on historical experience suggesting that full implementation of any of the key dimensions of SI will likely take a number of years. This assumption and the assumption about resources take a more instructional stance toward local collaborative efforts. While slightly more top-down in tone, these statements are still far from directing local collaboratives to make significant changes in their budgets or mandating any particular level of commitment.

While a design team with diverse membership produced the Markers, the members of this team all recognized some basic problems with the existing system of support for at risk families. Table 1 outlines some of these problems and references specific markers (see Table 2 for Markers) that are designed to address these problems.

The Markers of Progress presented in Table 2 are organized into four levels of SI which were originally delineated by Agranoff in 1991–the direct service level, the program level, the policy level, and the organiza-

TABLE 1. A Guide to System Risk Factors and Service Integration Responses to These Risks

System Risk Factor	Possible Service Integration Responses
No one agency is in charge of the well-being of children	Examine the organizational structure and responsibilities of the service collaborative and of the individual service agencies. Markers #: 25, 26.
Agencies establish programs that provide only limited and short-term benefits.	Examine the way agencies provide services and relate risk levels to service. Markers #: 1, 4, 16, 18.
Agencies are protective of turf rather than protective of the total well-being of children.	Examine the way consumers experience services, and how the designs of programs and policies lend themselves to unwanted competition and prevent beneficial types of collaboration. Markers #: 2, 3, 6-10, 19-23.
Agencies emphasize the number of clients served rather than the results achieved.	Explore how to pool program evaluation resources and establish protocols for joint accountability. Markers #: 13, 24.
Agencies operate under different mandates.	Explore possibilities for sharing resources so that each agency can both more effectively fill its mandate and improve the lives of children and families. Markers #: 10, 6, 20-23.
Agencies provide services on a reactive basis rather than a proactive basis	Explore how it might be possible to combine efforts and act more systematically in ways that allow more resources to be directed toward prevention. Markers #: 4, 5, 9.
Neither agencies nor the communities know the size of the universe that needs help.	Combine surveying and environmental scanning efforts. Markers #: 4, 10, 7, 8.
Service locations and procedures may hinder effective use of services	Examine how locations and procedures affect service use and plan for the appropriate response. Markers #: 5, 10, 20.

Source: Adapted from forthcoming monograph: Mendonza, Don. *Planning Strategies to Help Children Become Successful Adults: A Planning Manual.* Athens, GA: Carl Vinson Institute of Government, University of Georgia.

tional level. One of the key rationales for choosing to include a service integration marker in the instrument was that the marker be, as much as possible, something that is either visible itself or has components that are visible (i.e., can act as fairly indisputable markers of progress). Hence, evidence that service workers *feel* that they are not duplicating services is not considered concrete enough to indicate that duplication does not exist.

TABLE 2. Markers of Progress for Service Integration

SERVICE LEVEL

1. Holistic/Comprehensive

Family support efforts reflect holistic and comprehensive goals (i.e., family-determined goals not individual treatment goals or goals that are the result of a specific focus or concern of only one or a few agencies):

a. families and a full-spectrum of providers are involved in development of customized family plans;
b. confidentiality is not an issue;
c. when family goals logically demand family support services from collaborative partners (or others), the family support record will indicate that a good faith effort was made to link families to needed services;
d. the family begins to view the system as a resource.

2. Family-Driven:

Family plans and support services reflect family choices with respect to:

a. cultural values;
b. service provision sequence and timing;
c. preferred treatment modalities.

3. Efficient, Team Provision

Persons working with families do not duplicate each other's functions or services with respect to families that are common to more than one service provider:

a. the persons involved with a family know who else is involved;
b. some rule or mechanism exists that insures that duplication of effort, services, or functions does not occur (e.g., generic case managers or community services representatives who are hired, trained, and managed by the collaborative; or "the first agency to have contact with a family provides case management"; or "the agency with the highest priority service provides case management");
c. accessing resources that exist or are authorized and distributed in other agencies or facilities is no more difficult than accessing resources that are provided at a worker's home base;
d. confidentiality is not a barrier (i.e., because the family drives the process);
e. workers have a common understanding of their respective, non-overlapping roles in a family's plan;
f. workers are evaluated based on the degrees of support they give to an integrated, family-centered approach to helping persons in need.

TABLE 2 (continued)

4. Appropriate Scope and Scale of Effort:

Ideally:

a. all families entering the system would be screened for their needs related to integrated family support; and
b. all those who need and desire a particular level of support (e.g., those who are ready to make life changes and who are involved or likely to be involved with more than one agency) would be able to receive the appropriate degree of integrated support.

Triage rules for directing families to support are continually evaluated to insure: (a) the greatest effect for the cost and (b) consistency with community standards of equity.

5. Accessible Front-Line Workers/Information Resources

a. hours of availability make it convenient for families;
b. family support services are provided in places and facilities that are convenient for families and that involve the least wait and travel time;
c. workers display respect and common courtesy to families;
d. families can easily notify workers of a need (e.g., on an answering machine) and are able to speak to someone from a collaborative agency with X hours of notification;
e. information about the full spectrum of community resources is available at all collaborative facilities and important information is clearly displayed (e.g., office hours, etc.).

PROGRAM LEVEL

6. A Culture of Joint Program Planning, Administration and Budgeting

Partners meet for ___ amount of time for the purposes of making all agency program budgets more congruent with the collaborative's goals for families and children, including:

a. Identification of discretionary resources in all partner agency budgets (i.e., those available for joint programming).
b. Joint assessment of how categorical funds might better meet collaborative goals.
c. Agreement to design new programs jointly.
d. Joint evaluation and review of agency-specific programs in terms of their ability to advance collaborative goals/outcomes.

7. Common Intake

Consumer can apply and be given access to any service from any partner agency facility (e.g., Ga. Common Access form).

8. Common Family Needs and Strengths Assessment A generic, comprehensive family assessment is common across partner agencies.
9. Consistent Referral Families are directed correctly to resources the first time they enter the system.
10. Integrated Information Systems (assumes confidentiality and security will be maintained) a. Providers only enter information once. b. Referrals are automated. c. Information updates are shared. d. (fairly high) ___% of service providers have the system available to use. e. Managers can use the system to assess: 1. family needs; 2. availability, utilization and intensity of services provided to all members of a family over time (use a + b to identify gaps in service); 3. staff assignments and workloads; 4. referral patterns in relation to gaps.
11. Joint Purchasing
12. Joint financial management services among agencies.
13. Joint program evaluation and quality control services among partner agencies.
14. Consolidated personnel administration for partner agencies (e.g., related to recruitment, job classification and compensation, policies, etc.
15. Consolidated transportation systems for partner agencies.
16. Enactment of a **comprehensive, long-range facilities plan** that will be congruent with collaborative goals for multi-purpose, family-centered service delivery.
17. Comprehensive sharing of general resources (e.g., equipment, supplies, excess space, specialized skills, etc.).
18. Training Programs Support Flexible, Comprehensive, Preventive Services Training programs are assessed for how they fit with collaborative goals/outcomes, including: a. capacity of current workers to fulfill their role in this manner; b. amount of training needed in general per function to perform functional role in this manner; c. amount needed by specific workers in the community. A cross-training **plan is enacted** by the collaborative and resources are provided to implement the plan.
19. Staff and Management Assignments Support Integration at the Direct Service Level a. joint assessment of staff locations, service and management responsibilities; b. plan is enacted by collaborative to realign locations and responsibilities to better fit collaborative goals.

TABLE 2 (continued)

POLICY LEVEL

In general: Partner's Written Policies Support integration efforts at service and program levels: e.g., job descriptions and performance evaluations reflect an effort to create Effective Cross-Agency Teamwork or Partner's Written Policies Support Collective Management of Personnel and Staffing at shared, co-located, and joint program sites or confidentiality policies work to make integrated family support possible.

20. Streamlining of Services

a. policies support the conducting of a comprehensive streamlining analysis;
b. policies support using the analysis to develop strategies for eliminating redundancy of, and gaps in services and functions (e.g., application, assessment, eligibility, evaluation, etc.) and reducing consumer wait, travel time and other service barriers;
c. policies support integrated information system planning.

21. Financing

a. local agency policies support funding of integrated, family-focused services;
b. written agreements solidify commitment of all partner agencies to invest money earned from refinancing efforts into collaboratively-determined prevention/early intervention strategies;
c. collaborative has performed financial analysis to estimate the maximum refinancing potential of the community;
d. collaborative draws down monies at 85%+ of its potential.

22. Advocacy

a. partners conduct joint annual public awareness/advocacy campaigns congruent with the collaborative goals;
b. partners develop a joint advocacy effort and pool resources for lobbying, etc.;
c. collaborative makes comprehensive study of local policy barriers and develops barrier removal process.

23. Confidentiality

a. policies and practices are assessed to insure maximum level of service and information system integration while maintaining family dignity and choices.

24. Joint Accountability and Outcomes Evaluation

a. the collaborative publishes a service system report card outlining the connection between system-wide expenditures and policies and agreed-upon goals for families and children.

ORGANIZATIONAL LEVEL

25. Agencies Combine to Better Serve Families (typically involves state-level support).

Instead, the markers require that communities be able to point to a written rule or policy that (assuming it is followed) would insure that duplication did not frequently occur. In order to meet the visibility test, an attempt was made to break down the more abstract Markers into measurable components. These components can be assessed independently, and during the studying and consensus building phase, each component can be given a separate priority and feasibility rating.

At the services level, for example, the "holistic/comprehensive family support" marker has approximately five components that the development team believed to be integral to the marker, and to add a certain degree of visibility or measurability to the marker. For example, one can examine case records to see if they show evidence of whole-family, rather than individual, support goals (see Marker 1). These records would also indicate whether a full-spectrum of providers (i.e., sufficient to address the entire spectrum of family goals) have been involved in the development of the family support plan (see Marker 1-a). Similarly, when a goal logically demanded an effort to link the family with a provider of a specialized service, the case record would show that an effort was made in this regard (see 1-c). Interviewing or surveying the family and the providers involved would indicate whether confidentiality was a barrier issue in the effort to provide support (1-c), and interviewing families would tell one whether the family views the service system as a resource that has meaning and that provides benefit (1-d).

One of the more difficult sets of marker components to frame was the set associated with efficient, team provision of services (see Marker 3). In some descriptions of service integration efforts, it is assumed that there is "one best way" to integrate service personnel. This way might be to organize a group of community service representatives who broker services across agencies and who are responsible to the collaborative partnership rather than an individual agency. Generalized or generic family support workers are often described as operating in a similar organizational context. The efficient, team provision marker, however, does not assume that any particular way of organizing service delivery is best in all circumstances; it only requires that there be some way–such as a case allocation rule, a services review team, or a single organization taking responsibility–to insure that service providers do not duplicate or interfere with each other as they go about helping the same family (Marker 3-b). Establishing and implementing such a rule could require significant effort on the part of a collaborative. If a collaborative was not ready to take this step right away, it might nevertheless choose to set in place mechanisms that would at a minimum insure that the people involved with a family know who else is involved (i.e., Marker 3-a). Similarly, implementing Marker 3-c which would insure that a family support worker in one agency could access resources in another agency with the same ease as a worker in the agency where the resources are being drawn might be more difficult than developing a system where workers have a common understanding of their respective, non-overlapping roles in a family's plan. However, in some communities, achieving progress on the former might be much more meaningful than achieving progress on the latter.

Having a full range of service providing partners explore just how a marker is implemented can be important. For example, in one case it was discovered that even though some of the partners thought that confidentiality had ceased to be an issue because a cross-agency confidentiality waiver form had been created, other partners indicated that they were not aware of the existence of the form, while still other partners indicated knowing about the form but not using it consistently. In the exploration process, issues discovered in discussing a marker at one level can lead to a related marker on the same level or one on a different level. Discussing confidentiality issues at the service level, for instance, will often lead to a discussion of developing integrated information systems, a program level marker, that would tend to support a more automatic implementation of confidentiality protocols. During the development process, the design team worked from the service level up. As a result, choosing makers at this level often led to developing markers at the other levels that would logically support the service level marker. Obviously, some program and policy-level markers such as building integrated client information systems, use of common applications, common case assessments and referral procedures, and the streamlining of services to reduce consumer wait and travel time are likely to have a direct and immediate effect on family members' experiences of the service system.

Other markers did not logically emerge from a direct examination of how consumers experience the service system. Instead, these markers were included because the literature on and experience with organizational operations led the design committee to believe that achieving a marker could indirectly have a positive effect on the experience of consumers. Service integration markers that work indirectly also typically have their effect only in the long term. Such markers can be categorized into two groups: (1) cost-cutting, operational efficiency markers such as integrating agency back office operations (e.g., as purchasing, accounting, and personnel administration). And (2) program efficacy markers such as building a culture of joint program planning, administration, budgeting, and program evaluation. This latter group of markers are important indicators of a community's ability to establish joint outcomes accountability. That is, these markers indicate that agencies have ceded some of their autonomy related to program design to a collaborative partnership. (Obviously, the ceding of authority can only cover programs whose parameters are not mandated by law.) This is important because establishing joint accountability for outcomes will be meaningless if the partnership being held accountable is unable to affect the design of the system inputs. With markers such as Markers 6, 10, 13, 18 and 19 in place, it becomes possible to do such things as: shift resources away from the least effective programs and toward the more effective ones; redesign programs in line with research findings and collaboratively established goals; and pool the knowledge base of numerous program managers, planners, and evaluation specialists.

Although program level service integration efforts can substantially affect how families experience the service system, most program-level markers cannot be fully implemented without agency executives establishing policies permitting integration at lower levels in the organizational hierarchy. In this sense, each program-level marker can be thought of as having a parallel marker at the policy level. For conciseness, only some of these parallel markers are directly referenced in the policy level section of the Markers instrument. However, if one of the goals of a Markers of Progress facilitated process is to have policy makers review all the markers relevant to their level of responsibility, it would be important to include most of the program-level markers in this review. In addition to permitting and supporting specific program-level service integration efforts directly, policy makers can also nurture service integration in a few more general ways, specifically by setting up policies that support funding of integrated, family-focused services. Such policies might, for example, mandate that some or all of the new funds generated through refinancing of existing programs be invested in integrated rather than agency specific or category specific effort (see Markers 21-a, b). Other policies might insure that the collaborative use its resources and influence to maximize the refinancing potential of individual agencies so that the community as a whole benefits. While such a policy might seem odd, the experience in Georgia suggests that some agencies may not be taking advantage of their refinancing opportunities for any of a variety of reasons.

Finally, establishing policies to support streamlining efforts will be crucial (see Marker 20). Streamlining essentially involves an attempt to re-engineer processes that cut across agencies. Just as your garden variety, single-firm re-engineering effort requires support from those at the highest levels of the organization if it is to be successful, it is even more imperative that cross-agency streamlining efforts have this type of support. Policies are needed to deal with such issues such as how workers whose jobs have a potential for being redesigned will be involved in the process and how they will be treated when such decisions are made. Also, a number of service integration efforts will result in a rearrangement of agency workload, managerial prerogatives, organizational autonomy, and fiscal security. Some general policies and principles related to these issues need to be in place prior to going forward with some of the more ambitious service integration efforts. As an example, an SI committee at one local Family Connection site designing a one-stop services application process established a principle that no agency would be made worse off because of their willingness to take on responsibility for the using the form at their agency. This policy or principle then led to a program level effort to create a workload sharing formula for redistributing resources among agencies in cases where an agency experienced costs in excess of routine costs for completing applications for their own programs.

The last level of service integration makers is the organizational level. The major question at this level is whether or not the work of separate agencies would actually be performed better by a single unified agency. For some people, such organizational consolidation is the defining mark of service integration. Unfortunately, we know little about the circumstance in which consolidating agencies actually results in a marked improvement in the delivery of services. The record of this type of organizational level integration tells us that simply placing two or more agencies under one roof will not in and of itself insure any integration at the level where families can directly benefit–the service level. That consolidating services under one mega-agency has not been a panacea may be due in part to the large scale on which these efforts have traditionally been tried (e.g., at the state or national level). Although there may be reason to believe that consolidation would be more effective on smaller scale, most public human service agencies at this level, being creatures of the state, are denied this option. For this reason, people facilitating the Markers' process have tended to spend little time on the Markers this level.

Testing the Instrument: After a final draft of the Markers was developed, the Evaluation Committee of the Family Connection contracted with the Carl Vinson Institute of Government to test the Markers in a number of local FC sites. During the spring and summer of 1995, the Markers were used in a pilot process in four FC sites. Two of the sites were among the original 15 FC sites, one site had completed its year of planning and had begun implementation, and one site had just entered initial planning. The pilot of the Markers was designed to answer: (1) whether the SI markers (or areas of service integration) are relevant to the test communities; (2) whether the measures of progress (running across the top of the instrument) are adequate and appropriate for gauging progress; (3) how the instrument would best be used in communities at various stages of development; and (4) whether the Markers instrument is worth using.

The piloting process at the four sites typically involved a 10-15 minute introduction to the Markers, a large group discussion of how the instrument was designed, its purposes, and assumptions, how it might be used, and the meaning of particular markers. Following this discussion, participants were asked to break up into groups of four or five. The facilitator requested that the groups discuss each marker individually and attempt to choose one or two markers from each level that they believed their community should consider working on during the next two to three years. When the participants reformed into a large group an attempt was made to reach consensus as to priority Markers for the community. At the end of the session, participants were asked to evaluate the Markers instrument and process. Approximately forty local FC collaborative leaders participated in the piloting of the Markers instrument.

FINDINGS

The Markers: With respect to the markers (or areas of service integration), over 90% of the responding participants indicated that the markers were comprehensive, generally understandable, and relevant to their community and program. However, a few participants commented that some Markers may be unrealistic for certain size counties. It was also noted that some markers could use more explication and might need to be couched in layman's terms.

Because the design of the Markers followed Agranoff's four levels of SI, it was not surprising that a couple of participants noted a certain interrelatedness among certain markers. On the one hand, this interrelatedness could be confusing because of the seeming redundancy of markers on the different levels. For example, the issue of confidentiality is evident at the direct service, program, and policy levels. On the other hand, a good argument can be made that the potential barrier to improved services presented by excessive and counterproductive confidentiality restrictions is, in actuality, three interrelated but distinct barriers. For example, it is common for front-line human service workers in rural areas to report that confidentiality is not a barrier. When queried, however, one often discovers that official policies and program-level information systems may still present barriers to effective and systematic sharing of client information.

What typically occurs in rural areas is the establishment of informal worker-to-worker networks that essentially bypass official policies and systems. Hence, although confidentiality ceases to be a barrier to effective services as long as the informal network exists, when this network is disrupted either by personality conflicts or by changes in personnel, the issue of confidentiality-as-a-barrier will likely reemerge. Similarly, it may be possible to address the confidentiality issue at both the policy and direct service levels, but not at the program (or information system) level. In this case, confidentiality might not arise as a salient issue in everyday practice, but information sharing would also not likely occur to the degree that would facilitate best practice.

The pilot of the Markers process suggests that the rationale for the apparent redundancy in the Markers will probably need to be more fully explained. Alternatively, the process for working with the markers at the various levels could be structured so that the seeming redundancy became less visible to the participants. For example, if direct service workers were to address direct service level markers, program managers address program level markers, and agency executives address policy level markers, the seeming redundancy would be less obvious to the participants. This alternative process, however, has some disadvantages with respect to the potential for collaborative partners at different hierarchical levels being able to communicate with one another. The results of the FC first phase evaluation indicated, for example, that such cross-level communication was a major contributor to local collaboratives identifying and addressing barriers, especially policy barriers, to improved service delivery. One of the key strengths of having some services delivered by workers who are supervised by the collaborative as a whole, rather than by an individual agency, is that direct service workers appear to be more willing to speak their minds about service delivery problems across the spectrum of potential problems for a couple of reasons: (1) there is no established organizational culture that is tied to a unique service category, profession, or funding stream; and (2) there is no clear-cut hierarchy that can easily limit the subject matter for discussion or the channels for communications (O'Looney, 1992).

The Measuring Scale: As with the markers, the vast majority of the respondents to the Markers evaluation survey (> 95%) reported that the measuring scale being used (see Figure 1) to assess progress with respect to the individual markers (or areas of SI) was adequate and would be useful in helping the local collaborative chart progress over time. The pilot process, however, resulted in a couple of substantial improvements to the Markers instrument. First, it was suggested by a number of participants that when collaboratives begin to assess progress toward service integration within traditional mainline agencies that they list the specific organizations that had fully or partially implemented an SI marker. This listing, it was noted, would serve both to highlight the within-agency SI achievement and would help identify local expertise. Identifying organizations who have already reached an SI benchmark is important because the organization in question may be able to provide a model or starting point from which other collaborative partners and the collaborative as a whole can initiate SI efforts and activities. For example, at one site where the Markers process was used, it was discovered that one agency already had in place a comprehensive family assessment (as opposed to individual client assessments). Other agency representatives noted that they would be willing to use this agency's comprehensive family assessment form as the starting point for constructing a family assessment instrument that could be used by all partner agencies.

In addition to listing the organizations who were "early adopters" of particular SI markers, it was suggested that the date at which the marker was implemented at particular agencies or organizations be recorded. In this manner, it would be possible to assess the time it takes to move through the stages of progress from planning to SI pilot to implementation in mainline agencies. Ultimately, if such time-line data could be collected from a number of community collaborative sites, it might even be possible to begin to estimate the mean and minimum times for making progress with respect to certain markers. Such information would be particularly valuable in helping new collaboratives plan and budget for SI projects.

A second improvement to the measures component of the Markers instrument is related to how the collaborative partners are directed to go about choosing the SI markers they plan to work on in the near term. In the original draft, participants in the Markers process were only instructed to rate the priority they would give to each marker. In the revised instrument, it is recommended that participants discuss and rate both the priority level of the markers and the "feasibility" of implementing the marker. Discussions about priority appeared to help partners to identify the areas of service integration that would be most beneficial for the local community at that point in time, while discussions of feasibility seemed to assist partners in identifying and understanding the nature of the potential barriers to service integration. For many in the pilot study respondent group, the discussion of feasibility generated important insights into the nature of the specific opportunities and obstacles that were unique to that individual collaborative. Discussions of feasibility (of making progress on a marker) seem to help participants to focus in a concrete manner on who would support and who might stonewall the SI effort, if and where resources might be available, and what existing policies might present a barrier to implementing the SI effort.

To a certain degree, the discussions related to priority and feasibility provide a forum in which collaborative partners are encouraged to, first, raise questions about expected *benefit-cost* ratios of specific SI efforts, and secondly, to compare the benefit-cost ratios involved in achieving one SI marker versus another. Service integration entrepreneurs can gain strategic understanding from discussions of benefit-cost questions. They can then use this understanding to design more effective strategies for promoting SI. For example, in a discussion of the feasibility of a particular refinancing effort at one Family Connection site, it becomes apparent that the local health director is skeptical as to the ability of refinanced services to generate funds in excess of the administrative costs of the refinancing scheme itself. Because discussions of feasibility will typically evoke this type of information, it becomes possible for an SI entrepreneur to consider a number of courses of action: she might negotiate with the health director to agree to test out his theory on a small scale, or alternatively, she could choose to focus efforts on another area of service integration where there is less skepticism as to the net benefits that can be generated. However, as long as the health director's (or other partners') skepticism remains hidden, promoting particular SI efforts involves negotiating numerous invisible pitfalls.

Finally, the testing of the Markers instrument also resulted in a recommendation as to defining the meaning of "feasibility" in the context of the Markers' process. A number of participants struggled with how to define "feasibility." Does feasibility refer to: (a) being able to move one or two cells forward on the scale of achievement; (b) partially or fully implementing the Marker in the service pilot; (c) beginning implementation in mainline agencies; or (d) completely implementing the Marker in all partner agencies? The recommendation that emerged from the pilot was for feasibility to refer to the ability to reach a point where a marker has at least been implemented in two or more mainline agencies (i.e., gone beyond the Family Connection SI demonstration projects). However, communities could define feasibility in a different way if they so please. The important thing is for partners to talk about the same thing when they evaluate a Marker's feasibility.

The Process: The process for using the Markers that appeared to make the most sense for the participants in the Markers' pilot was to use the Markers in an annual or biannual retreat/strategic planning setting. Because the Markers provide a global-level catalog of potential SI activities from which partners are asked to choose a few on which to work, it was felt that more frequent use of the Markers would be unnecessary. Once the markers had been chosen, individual sites would need to construct a series of more detailed indicators of progress for each marker. In addition, it is helpful to work in small to medium sized, multidisciplinary, cross functional groups to arrive at a consensus on which markers to address in the near future.

Typical responses about the process included: "I feel that if the activity did not take place in a group, you may not get the interactive results. People may view as simply another survey" and "Group conversation gave insight to potential barriers and allowed for group agreement to how instrument will be interpreted for our collaborative."

Value of the Markers: Ninety-one percent of the respondents who participated in the Markers' pilot indicated that use of the instrument would be worthwhile. The remaining 9% of respondents indicated that they were not sure as to whether the instrument would be of substantial value in their community. The qualitative data suggests that the few individuals who were skeptical about the use of the instrument were chiefly concerned about the time that the Markers' process might take.

When responses of the three types of sites (original, new implementation, and planning) were compared, there was a slight tendency for the original site participants to rate the Markers' process as being less worthwhile than the planning or new implementation sites. Given that original sites' participants were more familiar with SI concepts and had undergone other facilitated processes related to collaboration and service integration, this finding was not unexpected. However, even in original sites, the Markers appear to have generated some new insights about needing to focus their service integration effort on a doable number of components and to have a task force champion some specific SI strategies. Also, exposure to the Markers seems to have been useful in orienting new partners to the SI focus of the Family Connection. The overall value of the Markers appeared to be highest in sites that had not already committed tremendous amounts of *time* and resources to implementing new service programs. For sites who had made such commitments, a concern about "*projectitis*," or the tendency to get so caught up in the details of implementing a specific program or service that system change goals are ignored, appeared to be on the mark. One indicator of such "projectitis" was the tendency for a few individual respondents at such sites to express a concern about taking time to plan for service integration (much less implement an SI feature). Although the Markers-document-as-evaluation-tool represents a certain level of expectation with regard to local sites moving toward more integrated services, the participants in the pilot of the Markers would frequently suggest the need for more *state leadership* to remove policy barriers to local service integration. For example, one site noted the existence of state school policy prohibiting the use of school buses to transport adults. In removing this barrier, one local partner argued, it would be possible to conduct more family-centered services and educational programs. In addition, state leadership needed to be more explicit in their expectations of the level of effort and expenditure directed at service integration vis-à-vis new services.

Evaluative Function of the Markers: Although the Markers grew out of the work of the FC Evaluation Committee, participants in the Markers pilot identified strategic planning sessions as the ideal settings for using the Markers for the first time, while recognizing that over a series of such planning sessions the Markers will naturally perform important evaluative functions. At the local level, participants in the Markers pilot indicated that the assessment function provided by the Markers would likely encourage local collaboratives to be more responsible for carrying through on the effort to integrate services. They also believed that use of the Markers would likely lead to the creation of special SI committees or task forces, for carrying out these responsibilities. In this respect, the Markers could be viewed as supporting the development of *local leadership* for SI efforts.

A NEW AGENDA FOR RESEARCH AND PRACTICE

At the level of state leadership, extensive and strategic use of the Markers as an evaluative tool is still uncertain. While there is a recognition that SI efforts need to be institutionalized and maintained over a long period of time if they are to be successful, there is also a fear that institutionalization may involve an unacceptable degree of top-down management of a process that has been traditionally defined as being bottom-up. Nevertheless, some of the Evaluation Committee members recognize that the benefits of such institutionalization may outweigh the risks. This is especially the case if it is discovered that mid-level managers are resisting SI efforts in large measure because they are skeptical about the *benefit-cost* ratio of SI. If this were found to be the case, a systematic plotting of SI progress among numerous communities statewide would be important because it would either confirm or eliminate such doubts about the benefits of SI. If, on the other hand, the Markers are only used as a self-assessment tool without some measure of standardization and aggregation across collaborative sites, there would not be a sufficient number of observations to begin to identify what is the average cost associated with addressing a particular SI marker. Producing such data, however, means that communities will need to use the Markers in a fairly consistent and continuous way and to link the Markers' assessment with budget data on the costs of SI efforts.

State level leaders who want to move local collaboratives toward more aggressive SI efforts must make a number of choices as to whether they believe this can best be accomplished in a top-down or bottom-up fashion. Currently, the Family Connection's Markers represent a rather light handed state level leadership effort to use an evaluation tool to address the least threatening barriers to SI. Because the Markers tool is presented as a self-assessment instrument, there is an underlying assumption that local leadership for SI exists and is willing to plan for and implement SI efforts–once the benign barriers of a lack of *time* and the lack of discrete *starting points* are overcome.

However, because the Markers development task group focused on these benign barriers, the Markers process is probably less effective in handling the potentially serious barriers to SI represented by: (a) the lack of willing leadership, (b) the lack of information on the cost-benefit ratio of SI efforts, and c) the threat of SI to staff status and security. The choice to structure the Markers process as a self-evaluation tool rather than as a top-down evaluation tool means that the Markers could very well be successful only as long as there exists a willing leadership who only need time and an SI focus to be successful.

One way to avoid erring on the side of using the Markers tool in a manner that is too much top-down or too much bottom-up would be to take a research and development (R & D) approach to using the Markers. Such an R & D approach would require patience, dedication and openness, but would offer opportunities to improve the Markers' process over time (Henry & Dickey, 1993). For example, before deciding on whether the Markers should only entail self-assessment or should involve more comprehensive cross-community assessments, it would be worthwhile to discover to what degree human service leaders really believe that SI will result in substantial net benefits or to what extent current service workers would be willing to work in newly configured jobs at new locations. Such preliminary research would likely advance our knowledge of how to strategically promote SI in particular settings. At the very least, it would inform the debate as to whether the SI movement will need more top-down support, as Sabatier's (1986) work suggests, or whether it can thrive only on bottom-up implementation practices as Elmore (1978) believes may be possible. More evidence of using an R & D approach to evaluating and planning SI efforts is needed before this debate will be settled.

In this regard, the Markers present both unique opportunities and challenges for researchers and administrators to gather data in the process of facilitating important system change work. For example, the Markers' process when combined with some individual surveys or focus group measurements can itself yield valuable information about how service consumers, managers, and executives view particular SI features in terms of service priority, feasibility, benefit-costs, and organizational threat. This opportunity is also a challenge to researchers to gather information in sufficient amounts so as to draw reliable conclusions and aid strategic planning without simultaneously overwhelming the system change work with time-consuming instrumentation.

Having action-oriented research inform practice will be particularly important and particularly challenging if we discover that service integration is being stymied by factors less benign than the *lack of time* or the *lack of the clarity of definitions* and *starting points*. If, for example, we were to discover that there is a strong current of skepticism about the *cost-benefit ratio* of SI among managers at a certain level or in certain agencies, how this information is processed will be of great consequence. Organizing the research-administration partnership collaboratively (i.e., across agency and hierarchial lines) could contribute in important ways to the processing of R & D data. Such an organization would be less likely to sweep unwanted findings under the rug, and it would also be motivated to insure that high standards in data gathering and analysis are maintained.

This case study has identified a number of barriers to the development of Georgia's Family Connection collaboratives and has reported on how the use of an instrument and process for marking progress toward service integration may work to address, and in some cases overcome, these identified barriers. Specifically, a pilot study of the use of the "Markers of Progress" in a number of local collaborative sites suggests that this instrument and process can help to: (1) define some specific starting points for SI efforts and break down the service integration concept into potentially "doable" components; (2) promote local consideration of the need to allocate time to SI efforts; (3) facilitate consideration of the local costs and benefits of engaging in any SI activity; and (4) provide a means by which state leaders can encourage local collaborative leaders to conduct a self-assessment of their progress toward service integration.

The pilot study did not provide evidence that the Markers process as currently conceived would substantially help address the less benign barriers of "skepticism about the benefit-cost ratios of SI efforts" and "concern about job security and status due to service integration changes." In part, this may have been because the pilot study process was a voluntary exercise rather than a required decision making process. As such, underlying skepticism about SI and concern about job status and security may not have been brought to the surface to the same degree they would have been if the discussions were to lead directly to serious, concrete, and detailed SI plans. A collaboratively organized, research-administration partnership will likely be needed if the Markers are to be used in the most effective manner to promote high-benefit service integration efforts. Overall, the participants in the pilot study indicated that the use of the Markers instrument would be "very worthwhile" in their community and would promote more effective and purposeful planning and self-evaluation. Whether the Markers instrument ought to be used in a more systematic, top-down manner to assess SI efforts across sites should depend on further research into the relative strength of each of the barriers to service integration.

REFERENCE NOTES

1. Also, unlike corporate leaders who are able to borrow money on the expectation that future revenue streams from expanded or improved operations will be large enough to repay current loans, human services leaders traditionally have not had such power or even the ready access to information that would enable them to chance such an investment strategy (Friedman, 1995). For example, even if it were to be shown that it is 1,000% more efficient to deliver services through a single generic and community-wide family case management system (rather than through a plethora of individualized case management systems), no human service agency could individually effect the change.

2. For example, Congress backed a small Services Integration Pilot Program. One reason for continued interest in services integration can be found in recent studies arguing that SI is likely to be an essential component in welfare reform efforts such as the "Learnfare" reforms attempted in Wisconsin (Ethridge, 1993) and in efforts to more effectively implement the education and training features of the JOBS program (Jennings, 1994). Additionally, private foundations such as the Pew Charitable Trusts and the Annie Casey Foundation have began to support SI efforts through research, technical assistance, and program development activities (Center for Assessment and Policy Development, 1993), while state government associations such as the National Governors' Association have supported educating state policy leaders in SI concepts and in the development of policy councils needed to facilitate SI at the state level.

3. There are some plans to also create an instrument designed to assess progress toward building "Community Capacity," or the ability of more natural helping systems and organizations to improve the lives of children and families.

REFERENCES

Agranoff, R. (1991, November/December). Human services integration: Past and present challenges in public administration. *Public Administration Review*, 533-41.

Bruner, C. (1991). *Thinking collaboratively: Questions and answers to help policy makers improve services for children*. Washington, DC: Education and Human Services Consortium.

Ellickson, R.C. (1991). *Order without law: How neighbors settle disputes*. Cambridge, MA: Harvard University Press.

Elmore, R. (1978, Winter). Organizational models of social program implementation. *Public Policy, 26*, 185-229.

Friedman, M. (1995). Outcome-based budgeting. Presentation at the Family Connection Annual Conference, August 8, 1995. Materials published by the Center for the Study of Social Policy, Washington, DC.

Gardner, S.L. (1992). Key issues in developing school-linked, integrated services. *The Future of Children, 2*(1), 85-94.

Gardner, S.L. (1995). Governance in human service collaboratives. Presentation at the 1995 Annual Family Connection Conference, Augusta, GA, August 6-8.

Gray, B. (1985). Conditions facilitating interorganizational collaboration. *Human Relations, 38*(10), 911-36.

Gray, B. (1989). *Collaboration*. San Francisco: Jossey-Bass Publishers.

Henry, G.T. & Dickey, K.C. (1993). Implementing Performance Monitoring: A Research and Development Approach. *Public Administration Review, 53*(3), 203-12.

Human Organization Science Institute. (May, 1990). *Evaluation of the Northampton County intake and case management demonstration project*. Villanova, PA: Villanova University.

Jennings, E.T. (1994). Building bridges in the intergovernmental area: Coordinating employment and training programs in the American states. *Public Administration Review, 54*(1), 52-60.

Jennings, E.T. & Krane, D. (1994). Coordination and welfare reform: The quest for the philosopher's stone. *Public Administration Review, 54*(4), 341-348.

Kagan, S.L. (1991). *United we stand: Collaboration for child care and early intervention services*. New York: Teacher's College Press.

Kagan, S.L. (1993). *Integrating human services: Understanding the past to shape the future*. New Haven: Yale University Press.

Kingdon, J.W. (1984). *Agendas, alternatives, and public policies*. Boston: Little, Brown.

Kraus, A. & Pillsbury, J. (1993). Streamlining eligibility and intake systems (Resource brief #6). Washington, DC: National Center for Service Integration.

O'Looney, J. (1992). Family connection: Year one evaluation. Athens, GA: Carl Vinson Institute of Government, University of Georgia.

O'Looney, J. (1993a). Re-designing the work of education. *Phi Delta Kappan, 74*(5), 375-81.

O'Looney, J. (1993b). Beyond privatization and service integration: Organizational models for service delivery. *Social Services Review, 67*(4), 501-34.

O'Looney, J. (1994). *Evaluating human services collaboration and integration at the state and local levels*. Athens, GA: Carl Vinson Institute of Government, University of Georgia.

O'Looney, J. (1996). *Re-designing the work of human services*. Westport, CT: Greenwood Press.

Sabatier, P. (1986). Top-down and bottom-up approaches to implementation research: A critical analysis and suggested synthesis. *Journal of Public Policy, 6*, 21-48.

Schorr, L.B. (1989). *Within our reach*. New York: Anchor Books.

Senge, P.M. (1990). *The fifth discipline*. New York: Doubleday.

Tjosvold, D. (1986). The dynamics of interdependence in organizations. *Human Relations, 39*(6), 517-40.

Reclaiming Community: An Integrative Approach to Human Services

Paul Adams, DSW
Kristine Nelson, DSW

SUMMARY. Taking the community rather than the service system as its starting point, a community-centered approach to service integration seeks to interweave formal and informal systems of care. Working as part of a community–negotiating and building partnerships with families, social networks, and organizations to change problematic patterns and mobilize resources–requires not only collaboration among administrators, but teamwork among front line staff. Team members need to share work, knowledge, and resources, while building collaborative relationships with their counterparts in other organizations, service users, and other residents. Ensuring congruence between new, integrative methods of practice and the way they are introduced and managed may require substantial changes in management behavior. "Resistance" is best understood in this context as feedback to management about its need to change. *[Article copies available for a fee from The Haworth Document Delivery Service: 1-800-342-9678. E-mail address: getinfo@haworth.com]*

Discussions of service integration usually focus on what professionals do, how they relate to each other, and how services should be organized.

Paul Adams and Kristine Nelson are Professors, Graduate School of Social Work, Portland State University, Portland, OR 97207-0751.

The work on which this article is based was supported in part by the Obermann Fund and the Center for Advanced Studies at The University of Iowa.

[Haworth co-indexing entry note]: "Reclaiming Community: An Integration Approach to Human Services." Adams, Paul, and Kristine Nelson. Co-published simultaneously in *Administration in Social Work* (The Haworth Press, Inc.) Vol. 21, No. 3/4, 1997, pp. 67-81; and: *Human Services Integration* (ed: Michael J. Austin) The Haworth Press, Inc., 1997, pp. 67-81. Single or multiple copies of this article are available for a fee from The Haworth Document Delivery Service [1-800-342-9678, 9:00 a.m. - 5:00 p.m. (EST). E-mail address: getinfo@haworth.com].

Indeed, there is much to be learned both from practitioners and managers of effective services and from attempts to translate their experience into the mainstream of the human services system. In reaction to a human services system that is unresponsive, stigmatizing, and ineffective there has been a ferment of experimentation in recent years. Practitioners in many fields, usually working in isolation from each other, have redesigned services and reshaped practice. Those who wish to reinvent services so as to make them less fragmented and reactive, more comprehensive, integrated, flexible, and responsive can draw on these natural experiments.

One of the hopeful aspects of the recent work on reinventing human services is, indeed, the interest in learning from and generalizing the experience and tacit knowledge of successful practitioners (both line staff and managers). Because these innovators, like jazz musicians, may be better at doing what they do than explaining it, practice tends to run ahead of theory (Smale, 1995). Schorr (1988) made an important contribution to the improvement and integration of education, health, and social services by describing examples of successful programs and drawing lessons from them for those who wish to redesign service systems. Going beyond description, in developing community social work and locality- or patch-based services in the United Kingdom, the National Institute for Social Work created a Practice and Development Exchange that enabled successful innovators to learn from each other and to consult with administrators seeking to develop integrated and responsive services (Smale, 1993; 1995).

Paradoxically, the study of successful integrative services points, however, to the need for a different starting place. All these examples involve a more or less fundamental change in relations between professionals and those who use their services, a shift that recognizes the strengths and capacities of families, social networks, and communities, and seeks to work in partnership with them. The community, rather than the service system, needs to be the starting point of analysis.

Decentering human services, shifting them from the center of the picture of which they are part, implies that the care and protection of children or elders or people with disabilities is a shared responsibility (Moroney, 1986) involving families, local communities, and the state. This more modest view of the role of services does not imply a narrow targeting of intervention on the most critical situations, a common response to budgetary constraint that leaves service providers in the center of a rescue drama. It should lead, instead, to a broadening of the conception of human services, as promoting and enhancing the development of families and communities, as well as responding to problems and deficits (Chapin Hall Center for Children, 1994). Neither is this an argument for pushing more of the burden on the shoulders of family caregivers, usually women, already suffering under the strain. Rather it supports a shift from a residual, crisis-oriented approach to one that works with families and communities to address shared concerns and promote healthy development. Such a system would provide people with a little help when they needed it, rather than waiting until their situation is desperate to make services available.

Starting with a perspective that decenters the relationship between professional and client while recognizing the central importance of other supports in families and communities, leads to a number of conclusions about professional practice, the service delivery system, and management of the change processes involved in reinventing human services.

DECENTERING

A community-centered approach to integrating services recognizes that professionals are not at the center of helping systems, that most of the caring and controlling in which social workers and other helping professionals are engaged is done by others–families, kin and neighborhood networks, informal groups, churches, schools, and other organizations. Formal human services, as Hadley, Cooper, Dale, and Stacy (1987) put it, "represent no more than a single strand in the complex web of relationships and services, formal and informal, statutory and non-statutory, which together provide care and control in the community. The overall effectiveness of provision depends not on one part of this network alone but on how well the whole is woven together" (p. 95).

In their role as change agents at various levels, community-centered social workers become involved with networks of family and kin, neighbors, churches, schools, and other agencies and organizations. They encounter patterns of interaction that are problematic to some or all of those involved. They assume in relation to them a position of marginality: they avoid either becoming enmeshed in the problem-perpetuating patterns they encounter or being marginalized–standing on the edge of the system unable or unwilling to intervene to change those patterns (Smale, 1995).

There is no assumption here that networks are always helpful or communities always supportive. On the contrary, the social work task arises from the attenuated or problematic nature of the network or community. As Smale (1995) argues, the problems that bring individuals and families to the attention of human service professionals may best be understood as the malfunctioning of a network of people. The social work task is to understand the patterns of interaction that generate or perpetuate problems that may involve multiple system levels (such as family, neighbors, school, and social service and juvenile justice systems) and to intervene to change them. An important aspect of the decentering of the professional-consumer relationship is the recognition that it is part of this larger pattern of interactions. Agencies and workers who are oblivious of this larger system and their own part in it may become part of the problem-perpetuating pattern (Imber-Black, 1988; Holder & Wardle, 1981).

PARTNERSHIP

Decentering the professional-client relationship implies building partnerships and collaboration. In family-centered services this has meant not only shifting from the individual to the family as unit of attention, but involving parents and caregivers as full partners in the design, delivery, and oversight of services (Cohen & Lavach, 1995). There is good research evidence that a partnership mode of helping, which engages and respects the strengths, resources, and creativity of service users, enhances people's sense of control over their own lives (Dunst, Trivette, Boyd, & Brookfield, 1994).

Involving service users and other local citizens in the design and delivery of services is fundamental to developing an integrated service system that is responsive to its neighborhood and community context, culturally competent, and empowering. This is true not only of parents of children with mental or physical disabilities, where there may be minimal social distance in terms of class or race between professionals and families, but also in child welfare settings where poverty is more likely to be a decisive influence and where parents' behavior is usually the "problem" precipitating professional involvement.

The move toward "user-led services" in the United Kingdom (Morris, 1994) and family or consumer involvement in the United States (Cohen & Lavach, 1995) has shown that the full partnership of family or community members, especially those with direct experience of services, is essential to changing the discourse of professionals. They bring an expertise about their own situation, about the experience of using services, and about the community that provides vital information to professionals. Explicitly or simply by their presence on advisory and governing boards, in case conferences, and in training sessions, they remind workers and managers of the mission and purposes of the agency, holding them accountable for their professional behavior. They discourage deficit-oriented and client-blaming discussions of families and their interactions with formal service systems. They enable professionals to see strengths and capacities in families and communities to which they may have been blind, and they help assure that services and programs are driven by the needs of families and communities rather than by funding or bureaucratic considerations.

There is a tendency to see the community only as a resource which the worker can use to supplement his or her repertoire of interventions, putting together a bag of resources from different places–a support group here, a helpful neighbor there–and presenting them to the consumer. Instead, changing the community itself is part of the task and the service user can be a contributor to this process. Professionals do not, in this approach, use informal networks for their purposes, but seek to enable and support social networks to help them function more effectively. In this sense, the community both has resources for addressing its concerns and is the locus of problem-perpetuating patterns of interaction. Bringing resources to bear from a range of sources and intervening to change destructive patterns may be part of the same process, as when a family that has been defined by neighbors and professionals alike as a problem for the community is enabled to take on a new role in solving a neighborhood problem. Holder and Wardle (1981) describe an example where not only concrete needs were met, but a whole pattern of relationships involving service users, other local people, and professionals was transformed.

One of the results of bringing community into the thinking and practice of human service organizations is that it enables them to see "clients" not only as users of services, consumers of resources, victims, or threats to the safety of the community or their children. It goes beyond recognition of the strengths, resources, and expertise that consumers can bring to bear on their own situations and on which the worker can build. A community-centered perspective points to the importance of recognizing the capacity of those formally involved with human services to *contribute* to the community (Adams & Krauth, 1995; Checkoway & Finn, 1992; Checkoway, Finn, & Pothukuchi, 1995; Smale, 1995; Swenson, 1995).

People previously seen only as objects of intervention and consumers of resources may have a significant capacity to contribute to the caring tasks of the community. Recognizing this potential has been a particularly important aspect of integrated, locality-based, community-centered human service teams, such as the Iowa Patch Project described below and its counterparts elsewhere in the United States, Canada, and the United Kingdom (Adams & Krauth, 1995; Adams, Alter, Krauth, St. Andre, & Tracy, 1995). Checkoway, Finn, and Pothukuchi (1995) also describe how a whole group of the population, youth in at-risk neighborhoods–typically seen as problems, victims, or perpetrators–may be engaged as contributors to the building of community.

Even such an awareness of the capacity of service users to be contributors, however, may be distorted by a professional-dominated view of community. The danger is that citizens may come to be seen as adjuncts or unpaid helpers who assist the professionals in their work. If the decentering of human services professionals is taken seriously, however, it involves recognition that the task of the professional is to find ways to join the community and be helpful to it in carrying out its work of caring for its members. This is most effectively done through teamwork with community members and other professionals.

TEAMWORK: THE PATCH APPROACH

"Service integration" has sometimes consisted of little more than co-location of agencies in neighborhood offices. This may be a first step in integrating services and making them more accessible, but it does not ensure that the services are experienced as integrated, responsive, culturally competent, flexible, or comprehensive. They may be geographically more accessible, but no less dominated by narrowly professional, categorical, fragmented practice. The promise of community-centered services is in the possibility of realizing more fundamental shifts, from reactive work to practice that is also preventive and proactive; from individual casework to work that includes networks and the community; from services at arm's length, driven by bureaucratic and funding considerations, to services close to the community and responsive to its needs (Hadley et al., 1987; Adams et al., 1995).

Realizing this promise depends on service integration at the front line. Smale and his colleagues (1988) argued on the basis of experience with community-centered service integration in Britain that a team is the smallest unit of staff that can engage in community social work. The knowledge of the community and its patterns of informal and formal care, the variation and breadth of the tasks involved, are beyond the capacity of any one practitioner. A team has the capacity to work at all points of the social work map, doing direct and indirect work, service delivery and change agent activity (Smale, 1995). It can share its knowledge, wisdom, and resources flexibly and quickly. Even within the constraints of court-mandated work in child protection and juvenile probation, it can move some of the distance from individual caseloads to a shared workload, including proactive work involving projects or activities that arise out of needs identified in the course of carrying out mandated work. Even when individual cases remain the responsibility of a single team member, she is able to bring to her work the shared knowledge of the community, the support of the team, and the fruits of prior work by the team, for example in initiating a support group or developing links with local schools and churches.

Such teams, Smale and his colleagues (1988) argue, can adopt a community-centered approach even when the rest of their agency or service system continues in a traditional mode. Experience in Britain, however, points to the importance of administrative and funding structures for the long-term survival of community-centered practice. Flexibility in the use of funds, through such approaches as decategorization and wraparound, are especially important in the United States where reactive, case by case intervention is built into many funding structures.

The Patch Project in Cedar Rapids, Iowa was an attempt, funded by a grant from the Administration for Children and Families, U.S. Department of Health and Human Services, to transfer key principles of the patch approach to locality-based, community-centered services from the United Kingdom to an American setting. Its purpose was to improve services to children and families by translating the principles of service integration into a different practice on the ground. Doing so involved the development of an interagency team of public service workers (including state child welfare workers, county homemaker, city housing inspector, juvenile probation officer), a community house worker, a team coordinator, a sometime service user and local resident, and social work student interns. The team had responsibility for a neighborhood, or patch, of about 10,000 residents, including all the child welfare work for the area. It continued after the expiration of the federal grant in 1994 as an important part of the development of family resource centers in the county and of the process of decategorizing child welfare and juvenile justice funding streams.

The project demonstrated the feasibility of integrating services through a neighborhood-based, co-located interagency team of human service workers, representing both public and private non-profit agencies, without a large input of new resources. This approach to practice and service delivery mitigates problems of fragmentation, deficit- and crisis-orientation, bureaucratic rigidity, turfism, and the substitution of formal for informal systems. It promotes an interweaving of formal and informal resources, consumer and citizen involvement, prevention and early intervention, accessibility, and collaboration. It does this, not as an adjunct to existing services, but as a process of changing relations among agencies and between them and the communities they serve.

The project is described and assessed elsewhere (Adams et al., 1995; Adams & Krauth, 1995). Its significance for this discussion lies in the lessons to be drawn for administration of service integration efforts and the management of the change processes involved. These confirm in a U.S. setting the British experience with community social work.

DEVOLUTION OF DECISION-MAKING

There is in human services a parallel process whereby the powerlessness often experienced by families in face of a bureaucratic and threatening human services system is reproduced in the disempowered line worker whose capacity to use professional judgment or even common sense is tightly circumscribed by mandated procedures, rules, and regulations. Even senior managers feel themselves helpless in face of shrinking and unpredictable budgets, rising caseloads, and hostile public and media scrutiny.

Moving to a community-centered integration of services requires a reversal of this process. It means empowering workers to empower families, allowing and facilitating those working directly with families and communities to make more of their own decisions (Adams & Krauth, 1994). The key task of management is to provide space, the room to maneuver so that the human services team can develop its relationships with and knowledge of the community, form partnerships, and take initiatives on the basis of their own strengths and capacities and of the needs and strengths they identify as a result of their work in the community.

This involves learning from the team what barriers stand in the way of their work and finding ways around them. Moving toward a common approach to a shared workload requires much more role flexibility than is common in public or private agencies that depend on categorical funds and contracting for specific services on a case by case basis (Hadley et al., 1987). Decategorization of funding streams may be especially helpful in increasing a team's flexibility and capacity to respond proactively to community needs. More generally, the potential of service integration depends on flexibility at the local level in determining service delivery, financing, and management strategies, allowing workers to circumvent categorical restrictions and to be accountable for effecting change in partnership with families (National Center for Service Integration, 1994). Workers need to be empowered by management that is itself empowered by authoritative community service planning and governance structures that make it possible to recombine existing resources and restructure service patterns (Farrow, 1991; Melaville & Blank, 1991). The flexibility sought by interagency collaboratives at the management level can promote community-centered practice if it is extended to staff teams in the form of increased discretion to allocate their resources and time in the way best suited to addressing their tasks, maintaining a focus on change processes and results rather than procedures.

This approach stands in contrast to the market mechanisms and competition among providers praised by the advocates of "reinventing government" (Osborne & Gaebler, 1992). These have become, not a solution to the fragmentation, excessive paperwork, and stigmatizing of the human services, but a major part of the problem. Public sector workers find themselves rapidly plugging customers into services like an old-fashioned telephone operator connecting callers. They may buy for their customers a given number of hours of therapy from a private provider who has an incentive to provide those hours of service whether all of them are needed or not. No one under this system has an incentive to be proactive or to develop informal collaboration with other organizations such as schools, churches, or neighborhood groups. Rather than bringing an entrepreneurial spirit into the public sector, market reforms such as privatization and the purchase of services system have spread distrust, excessive paperwork, and fragmentation into the private and voluntary sectors that depend on government contracting for their income (Adams & Krauth, 1995).

Community differs from both bureaucracy and market as a direction for integrating services. A community-centered social work team sees those it works with not as customers to be served but as fellow citizens and community members with whom human service professionals can exchange ideas, concerns, and resources as they share responsibility for the community. Thus, instead of conducting focus groups as a kind of consumer research to learn what services were wanted, the Iowa patch team followed the example of an earlier social services team in London. Invited to participate in exchange meetings, local people joined team members in discussing both common concerns and the resources that citizens and professionals alike could bring to bear in addressing them (Adams et al., 1995).

Partnership of this kind involves negotiation of shared responsibility for addressing common concerns. A community-centered team is constantly engaged in negotiating care in the community, whether at the level of individual families or the provision of a wider service (such as a summer recreation program), or working to improve interactions among families, schools, and the child welfare system. Service integration cannot from this perspective be mainly a matter of negotiation among administrators. If it is, the result is likely to be a host of additional meetings for overburdened managers without an appreciable impact on the services that citizens experience.

Partnership implies a devolution of responsibility as close to those actually involved in the helping process as possible. Line workers and social service teams cannot negotiate in good faith with families, other workers and agencies, or others involved in the social context, if they find they are continually countermanded by managers higher up the organizational hierarchy. The effect will be disempowering for workers and others involved and the result is likely to be cynicism and distrust (Smale & Tuson, 1993; Adams & Krauth, 1994).

MANAGING CHANGE, CHANGING MANAGEMENT

Translating service integration into a different front-line practice and a different relationship between professionals and community requires fundamental changes in the relations between managers and workers. It is common when attempting to promote a new approach to delivering services for administrators to define implementation problems at the line level as "resistance." This view reinforces a deficit orientation to staff that the reform itself may be attempting to remove in relation to service users.

Such a reaction on the part of workers may be better seen as feedback either about the innovation itself or about the need for management to be more creative in introducing it. For example, a major concern among line workers burdened with rising caseloads and shrinking resources is that a new way of working simply adds to their work without providing additional resources. Managers themselves may see an innovation such as patch as an add-on to existing services rather than as a different way of doing the existing business of the organization. At first, management in Iowa thought that nothing would change other than the location of the workers. Workers too saw the development of partnerships in the community as another task to be accomplished in addition to their mandated work. Over time, however, both workers and managers came to see community-centered practice not as an add-on, but as a different way of accomplishing the work of their agency.

Generally, community-centered workers aim to build the caring capacity of the people and networks involved, rather than substitute for them. By building partnerships with families and their networks, with agencies, schools, churches, and neighborhood groups, they and their team help interweave formal and informal caring (Bayley, Seyd, & Tennant, 1989). They spend less time doing to or for families and more time working with them, less time on crisis intervention and more on prevention and early identification (Adams & Krauth, 1995).

As with a kaleidoscope, the aim is to rearrange the pieces rather than add new ones. If workers are successful they may reduce their formal caseloads significantly while increasing their informal work, as happened in the United Kingdom (Hadley & McGrath, 1984). In that case, it is important that workers know they will not be punished for their success by losing staff to less successful areas with higher caseloads. It may also be important, as it was for the patch team in Iowa, for them to receive formal acknowledgement of their proactive and informal community work, especially if other workers and supervisors see only their declining caseloads.

"Resistance" may also point to a lack of congruence between the innovation being introduced and the method of its introduction. Innovations that devolve responsibility to line staff need to allow staff themselves room to be creative in their adaptation to the context they know. Otherwise, managers put staff into a double bind by ordering them to be spontaneous. They reinforce, rather than reverse, the disempowerment of line staff, which is then reproduced as disempowering practice with families.

Managers (and policy makers) need to be clear that complex innovations requiring flexibility and creativity from front line staff have to be reinvented in each local context. This involves replication of concepts rather than of program details (Finney, 1993; Schorr, 1993). Changes that by their nature have to be negotiated with local people in specific communities cannot be imposed by administrative fiat (Martinez-Brawley, 1995).

Idaho's statewide reform of its child welfare system to promote family preservation and family-centered principles illustrates the changes in philosophy and practice necessary to transform current fragmented systems into an integrated family-centered system. The same principles would apply to developing a system of proactive, locality-based, community-centered, interagency teams (Nelson & Allen, 1995).

In 1985, Idaho's poor performance on a compliance audit for the Adoption Assistance and Child Welfare Act of 1980, precipitated a gradual shift from a "rescue" based child protection and juvenile justice system to a family-centered model. Deciding to pursue system-wide reform rather than to add family preservation as another categorical program, the state integrated child protective, juvenile justice, child mental health, JOBS, adoption, and substance abuse services into a single practice model with a common administrative structure (Patterson, 1992).

Seeking to redirect and retrain existing staff, Idaho decided on a "bottom-up" process of change that engaged the creativity of line staff as well as management. Treating staff the same way they are expected to treat families, the agency sought to recognize and respect the strengths and values of individuals and their ability to grow and change. Management valued staff input and tolerated mistakes without instilling fear of punishment. In keeping with the collaborative relationships throughout the system, administrative reviews of local offices were directed toward solving problems and improving practice rather than enforcing procedures. Although required only every 18 months, local offices often requested reviews more frequently (DHHS, 1991). Management involvement is seen by staff as "helping to get us better at what we are supposed to be doing" rather than as intrusive or hierarchical (DHHS, 1991, p. 34).

In addition, increased involvement in treatment teams of other service providers led to a sharing of clinical skills, innovations, and successes and of responsibility for the risks inherent in family preservation. Schools, police, churches, other agencies, and natural helping systems also assisted communities to overcome their initial perception that the agency was abandoning its responsibility to protect children (Patterson, 1992). Whenever possible, the suggestions of community-based advisory groups, including advocates and consumers, were implemented and full explanations were provided if they were not (DHHS, 1991).

Idaho's experience points to the importance of a parallel process in which the way change happens models the changes sought. It illustrates the advantages of a bottom-up process of change that enables agencies to incorporate staff knowledge and experience into policy development. Common features of the reforms described above are the capacity to learn from line workers' best practice and to allow changes in practice to precede administrative changes in rules and procedures. It was more than a year, for example, before the arrangements that set a team in motion in a Cedar Rapids, Iowa neighborhood were formalized in a signed interagency agreement. In Idaho, the system was allowed to evolve for several years before changes were codified in manual form. Many procedures including payment systems, caseload standards, work hours, and supervision methods were radically modified. This developmental, continuous learning approach enabled the system to draw on front line experience to increase flexibility and partnership with consumers.

CONCLUSION

If we start the discussion of service integration with the service network, which we hope to make less fragmented and crisis-oriented, more responsive and comprehensive, there is a danger of focusing on the problems of interagency collaboration as if the issue were entirely one of how the professionals organize themselves to deliver services to clients or consumers. The latter remain as objects of professional or bureaucratic attention, at best customers or consumers rather than full partners in and contributors to the process of change. Service integration then gets reduced to decentralization and co-location without necessarily changing the experience of families or front line workers.

An alternative starting point is the community of which formal human services constitute one element in the care and protection of its members. We have argued that starting with the community (a community-centered approach) implies decentering the professional-client relationship and building partnerships at all levels between helping professionals and community. This requires teamwork among workers able to share work, knowledge, and resources with each other, while building collaborative relationships with other agencies and organizations, and with service users and other residents. Bringing about these changes in the practice of line staff and their relations with families and the community may require, among other things, changes in management practice, so that there is congruence between the changes sought and the methods of introducing and managing them.

At the same time, community-centered practice requires line staff to take ownership of their team's development and strategy, to participate more than they are used to in managing their joint work. This has implications for team development, which, as Smale (1993) points out, "refers not only to developing the relationships between team members to further the integration of their work, but it also covers the development of shared work in areas of collective responsibility, such as the identification of area needs and resources and other functions" (p. 93). Building interorganizational and professional capacity to work effectively in a partnership mode is an ongoing process of learning and adaptation. Since teams and team-building are essential to this approach, training and consultation for practitioners and managers need generally to be provided on-site to teams of workers and/or managers rather than in the customary pattern of sending individual workers or managers to workshops (Hadley, Dale, & Sills, 1984).

Essential to developing community-centered integrated services is the involvement of local citizens and service users at every level as full partners in the design, delivery, and oversight of services. This includes case planning for services to their own families, team project development, staff training, and governance of interagency collaboratives. Effective interweaving of formal and informal care in the community also requires that social work agencies involve themselves at every level in the life of the community. It requires learning continuously about how care is being provided in families, social networks, and other formal and informal organizations, seeing how social workers and their agencies are themselves part of these patterns, and forming and reforming partnerships at all levels in the shared work of building the caring capacity of the community.

REFERENCES

Adams, P. et al. (1995). *Strengthening families and neighborhoods: A community-centered approach.* Final report on the Iowa Patch Project. Washington, DC: U.S. Department of Health and Human Services, Administration for Children and Families.

Adams, P., & Krauth, K. (1995). Working with families and communities: The patch approach. In P. Adams & K. Nelson (Eds.), *Reinventing human services: Community- and family-centered practice.* New York: Aldine de Gruyter.

Adams, P., & Krauth, K. (1994). Empowering workers for empowerment-based practice. In P. Nurius & L. Gutierrez (Eds.), *Education and research for empowerment practice.* Seattle: School of Social Work, University of Washington.

Bayley, M., Seyd, R., & Tennant, A. (1989). *Local health and welfare.* Aldershot, UK: Gower.

Chapin Hall Center for Children. (1994). *Children, families, and communities: A new approach to social services.* Chicago: Chapin Hall Center for Children at the University of Chicago.

Checkoway, B., & Finn, J. (1992). *Young people as community builders.* Ann Arbor, MI: Center for the Study of Youth Policy, School of Social Work, University of Michigan.

Checkoway, B., Finn, J., & Pothukuchi, K. (1995). Young people as community resources: New forms of participation. In P. Adams & K. Nelson (Eds.), *Reinventing human services: Community- and family-centered practice.* New York: Aldine de Gruyter.

Cohen, R., & Lavach, C. (1995). Strengthening partnerships between families and service providers. In P. Adams & K. Nelson (Eds.), *Reinventing human services: Community- and family-centered practice.* New York: Aldine de Gruyter.

Department of Health and Human Services. (1991). *Child welfare services program review: Idaho, Region X.* Washington, DC: DHHS.

Dunst, C.J., Trivette, C.M., Boyd, K., & Brookfield, J. (1994). Help-giving practices and the self-efficacy appraisals of parents. In C.J. Dunst, C.M. Trivette, & A.G. Deal (Eds.), *Supporting and strengthening families. Volume 1: Methods, strategies and practices.* Cambridge, MA: Brookline Books.

Farrow, F. (1991). Services to families: The view from the States. *Families in Society: The Journal of Contemporary Human Services, 5*, 268-276.

Finney, G.S. (1993). *Building from strength: Replication as a strategy for expanding social programs that work.* Philadelphia: The Conservation Company.

Hadley, R., Cooper, M., Dale, P., & Stacy, G. (1987). *A community social worker's handbook.* London: Tavistock.

Hadley, R., Dale, P., & Sills, P. (1984). *Decentralising social services: A model for change.* London: Tavistock.

Hadley, R., & McGrath, M. (1984). *When social services are local: The Normanton experiment.* London: Allen & Unwin.

Holder, D., & Wardle, M. (1981). *Teamwork and the development of a unitary approach.* London: Routledge & Kegan Paul.

Imber-Black, E. (1988). *Families and larger systems: A family therapist's guide through the labyrinth*. New York: Guilford.

Martinez-Brawley, E.E. (1995). Knowledge diffusion and transfer of technology: Conceptual premises and concrete steps for human services innovators. *Social Work*, *40*(5), 670-682.

Melaville, A.I., & Blank, M.J. (1991). *What it takes: Structuring interagency partnerships to connect children and families with comprehensive services.* Washington, DC: Education and Human Services Consortium.

Moroney, R.M. (1986). *Shared responsibility: Families and social policy*. New York: Aldine.

Morris, J. (1994). *The shape of things to come? User-led social services*. London: National Institute for Social Work.

National Center for Service Integration. (1994, Winter). Providing comprehensive integrated services for children and families: Why is it so hard? *NCSI News*, 1-3.

Nelson, K., & Allen, M. (1995). Family-centered social services: Moving toward system change. In P. Adams & K. Nelson (Eds.), *Reinventing human services: Community- and family-centered practice*. New York: Aldine de Gruyter.

Osborne, D., & Gaebler, T. (1992). *Reinventing government: How the entrepreneurial spirit is transforming the public sector*. Reading, MA: Addison-Wesley.

Patterson, K. (1992, Spring). Investing in an agency's "work family": Idaho's experience in implementing a family-centered practice model. *Prevention Report* (Newsletter of the National Resource Center on Family Based Services), 6-7.

Schorr, L.B. (1988). *Within our reach: Breaking the cycle of disadvantage*. New York: Anchor/Doubleday.

Schorr, L. (1993, June 16). Keynote address. In National Association of Social Workers, *Effective strategies for increasing social program replication/ adaptation*. Washington, DC: National Association of Social Workers.

Smale, G.G. (1995). Integrating community and individual practice: A new paradigm for practice. In P. Adams & K. Nelson (Eds.), *Reinventing human services: Community- and family-centered practice*. New York: Aldine de Gruyter.

Smale, G.G. (1993). The nature of innovation and community-based practice. In E.E. Martinez-Brawley (Ed.), *Transferring technology in the personal social services*. Washington, DC: NASW Press.

Smale, G., & Tuson, G. (1993). *Empowerment, assessment, care management and the skilled worker*. London: Her Majesty's Stationery Office.

Smale, G., Tuson, G., Cooper, M., Wardle, M., & Crosbie, D. (1988). *Community social work: A paradigm for change*. London: National Institute for Social Work.

Swenson, C.R. (1995). Professional understandings of community: At a loss for words? In P. Adams & K. Nelson (Eds.), *Reinventing human services: Community- and family-centered practice*. New York: Aldine de Gruyter.

Collaboration: A Study of a Children's Initiative

Anita S. Harbert, PhD
Daniel Finnegan, PhD
Nancy Tyler, MSW

SUMMARY. In times of shrinking resources within the social services, collaboration is being promoted as a more efficient way of meeting the needs of children and families. A study of a children's initiative collaborative developed to address the problems of children is reported. The authors present and use an evaluation framework which incorporated the dimensions of context, process, and outcomes of collaboration. The findings, based on the initial two years of collaborative effort, suggested the membership of the group and the process and structure governing the group's operations impacted the process and outcomes of the collaboration. *[Article copies available for a fee from The Haworth Document Delivery Service: 1-800-342-9678. E-mail address: getinfo@haworth.com]*

BACKGROUND AND PURPOSE

In the past decade, the needs of children in this country have surfaced as a major concern. Children and youth have been identified as at risk and losing ground on a number of fronts, including incidence of poverty, inade-

---

Anita S. Harbert is Director, Daniel Finnegan is Assistant Professor, and Nancy Tyler is Research Assistant, School of Social Work, College of Health and Human Services, San Diego State University, San Diego, CA 92182.

[Haworth co-indexing entry note]: "Collaboration: A Study of a Children's Initiative." Harbert, Anita S., Daniel Finnegan, and Nancy Tyler. Co-published simultaneously in *Administration in Social Work* (The Haworth Press, Inc.) Vol. 21, No. 3/4, 1997, pp. 83-107; and: *Human Services Integration* (ed: Michael J. Austin) The Haworth Press, Inc., 1997, pp. 83-107. Single or multiple copies of this article are available for a fee from The Haworth Document Delivery Service [1-800-342-9678, 9:00 a.m. - 5:00 p.m. (EST). E-mail address: getinfo@haworth.com].

quate health care, quality of education, employment opportunities, exposure to crime and drug abuse, etc. (Children's Defense Fund, 1992; Edelman, 1987; Grubb & Lazerson, 1983; Schorr, 1988; Sidel, 1986). Across the nation, a number of efforts are underway to turn the tide on the rapidly declining quality of life of America's children and youth. State and national initiatives have begun to address this problem. Examples of such efforts include the Coalition for America's Children and the Georgia Campaign for Children. A major theme which has emerged from these efforts is that with limited resources, different approaches are needed to resolve the difficulties confronting service providers in their efforts to respond to the needs of children and families (Kammerman, 1989; Scales & Brunk, 1990; Schorr, 1988; Steiner, 1981; Zimmerman, 1989). An assumption which underlies many of the current efforts is that systematic change is required to bring about a better means of serving children and families, and that such change can occur through interagency collaboration.

The social service delivery system in the United States and in other parts of the world are generally composed of a myriad of categorical programs, each designed to provide a specific service for categories of the population (Alaszewski & Harrison, 1988; Flynn & Harbin, 1987). At different points in time during the past few decades, attempts have been made to integrate or coordinate services among these categorical programs. Rein (1970) identified three types of problems which manifest themselves, given the current categorical system of social service delivery. These include the dispersal of similar functions, discontinuity of related functions, and incoherence when different functions are pursued without relationship to each other. Interagency service coordination, integration, or collaboration are general concepts used to describe a variety of efforts to reform the existing delivery system of categorical social services. Some researchers (Flynn & Harbin, 1987; Kagan, 1991) maintain that claims of the efficacy of interagency coordination and collaboration are based more on philosophical belief than on hard evidence.

Collaboration has resurfaced in the social service arena among human service, government, and community organizations as a better means to meet the needs of clients. Collaboration is being promoted, for it is believed that cost efficiencies can be achieved through joint delivery of similar services (Zald, 1969). It is also possible that through collaborative efforts, services can be made more accessible and provide better service to people who need assistance with complex problems (Gage, 1976). A report from The McKnight Foundation maintained that:

> Collaboration results in easier, faster and more coherent access to services and benefits and in greater effects on systems. Working

together is not a substitute for adequate funding, although the synergistic efforts of the collaborating partners often result in creative ways to overcome obstacles. (Mattessich & Monsey, 1992, p. 6)

THE CHILDREN'S INITIATIVE

In 1991, a concerted effort was initiated in a large metropolitan area in the Southwest United States to identify and address the status of children and families in the region. Spearheaded by the United Way, service providers in the area were gathered together to discuss the needs and problems confronting children and families. Subsequently, a comprehensive needs assessment was conducted on the status of children from prenatal through 18 years of age. As part of the needs assessment, data were collected on the status of children related to health, safety, and economic security; social service; education; physical fitness; social development; and employment and job training of youth. Community forums were held in an attempt to identify the priority needs of children and families. As a result of these forums, three basic needs were identified: (a) safer neighborhoods and communities, (b) quality education, and (c) a drug-free environment.

A major finding of the needs assessment maintained that existing resources were going to remedial services as opposed to preventive efforts. A conclusion of the assessment was that the reality of maintaining basic services, while at the same time attempting to create a service delivery system that will focus on prevention and early intervention, requires a new approach which uses available scarce resources more effectively.

In an effort to address the problems and priorities identified by the needs assessment, several foundations and organizations in the community committed funds and staff support to promote a Children's Initiative. The goal of the Initiative was to mobilize social service providers and citizens at large to address the needs of children. To launch the Initiative, a Steering Group, made up of representatives from the five funding organizations, began to work in 1992 to operationalize the Children's Initiative. This group identified a vision, a mission for the Initiative, categories of needs to be addressed, and the social service delivery systems to be affected. It was decided that the major thrust of the Initiative should be to create systemic change in service delivery systems and programs which serve children and families. It was also assumed that systemic change could best be put into effect through interagency collaboration aimed at long-term problem resolution which would direct existing resources to prevention and early intervention. The fields of service to be affected were health, education, safety, and economic security.

Once the parameters of the Initiative were identified, the Steering Committee created a Strategic Action Committee (SAC) composed of representatives from the target fields of service agencies and others able to create an overall plan for system re-design. The Committee's goal was to identify areas of service provision to be improved through interagency collaboration and interventive methods to better serve the needs of children and families in the area.

Since nothing of this magnitude had been attempted before in the area, an effort was made to study this collaborative effort. The literature suggested that the interagency collaborative aspects of the Initiative would manifest itself in three phases: the formative phase, aimed at obtaining collaborative agreement for a common vision on the part of the Strategic Action Committee in the four target fields of service; a developmental phase in which a strategic action plan for achieving that goal was designed; and the implementation phase when the action plan is carried out. This study focused on the formative phase of the Children's Initiative Collaboration. It attempted to identify those dimensions which influenced the collaborative development of a strategic action plan which would be used to implement a Children's Initiative.

Evaluating Interagency Collaboration

The literature suggests that evaluation of interagency collaboration is a challenging endeavor, fraught with many difficulties. Guthrie and Guthrie (1991) note that very often people do not think of evaluation of programs or collaborative efforts until they are well underway and it is too late to gather the necessary data. They stated that in this type of evaluation evaluators ask both summative and formative questions and go beyond traditional measures of program effectiveness. Kagan (1991) maintained that there is mounting literature that demonstrates the challenges of evaluating collaboration. She further stated that work has emerged that suggests collaborations are effective catalysts for change and much can be learned from their processes. Kagan identified a number of questions that should be assessed in this type of evaluation. For example: What differences does collaboration make? How do we know when we have achieved success? What have we really learned from pioneering efforts? Guthrie and Guthrie (1991) identified questions such as: How effective was the collaboration? Was communication improved? Have bureaucratic barriers been overcome? How can interagency collaboration be improved?

Flynn and Harbin (1987) discussed design issues that must be considered when conducting evaluations. They suggested consideration be given to the purpose and the audience; the framework that is selected, making sure that it is in conjunction with the paradigm; how the results will be used (summative vs. formative); research strategies (qualitative vs. quantitative); how the evaluation will be funded; and who should conduct the evaluation.

Kagan (1991) indicated that to assess the efficacy of collaboration, three conditions must be met: the goals of the endeavor must be clear, the collaboration must be implemented, and the standards of measurements must be precise and replicable. Many challenges exist to this type of evaluation including questions on how to define the goals of collaboration. Current research suggests two broad goals of collaboration–one relates to producing direct changes in service delivery systems; the other relates to fostering or creating systems change. Some collaborations may attempt both of these goals simultaneously.

Additional dimensions that make evaluations difficult arise because collaboration has multiple process and outcome dimensions, thus complicating the challenges of defining precise success criteria. For example, does success mean that all or part of the goals have been achieved? Or does overall success mean partial success in all areas or full success in a few areas? Kagan (1991) concluded that rather than seek overall indices of success or dubbing efforts as exemplary models, one may do well to consider partial conditions of success within specific circumstances. In addition, she indicated that evaluation is difficult because implementation is never fully completed; therefore, it is hard to attribute outcomes to a certain intervention if it cannot be determined whether the intervention has actually been implemented.

The second factor defined by Kagan (1991) is equally problematic. In order to attribute outcomes to an intervention, it is necessary to ascertain whether the intervention has been implemented. As collaborations are designed to be flexible and to meet changing needs, their implementation is never complete. Consequently, precise definition of implementation does not exist because it is a highly idiosyncratic and mutable condition. Moreover, the strength of collaborations is that they are tailored to meet changing local circumstances.

As one surveys the literature on evaluation of interagency collaboration efforts, two problems emerge. One problem relates to the fact that it is not always clear what type of interagency interactions are being studied. The other problem is the lack of a definitive framework for evaluating this type of interagency effort. Although researchers agree that multiple dimensions, rather than singular dimensions, contribute to the outcomes of such interorganizational efforts, they have yet to reach a consensus on the specific dimensions which may influence outcomes in order to address these problems. For purposes of this study, a working definition of collaboration and a framework for evaluating collaboration are provided below.

A Working Definition

Several researchers commented on the fact that defining collaboration is made complex by the ambiguities in practical usage and scholarly disagreements about the term. According to Swan and Morgan (1991), the term collaboration in practice is often interchanged with the terms integration, linkages, networking, cooperation, and coordination. In an effort to be more precise, Mattessich and Monsey (1992) provided a working definition of collaboration as "a mutually beneficial and well-defined relationship entered into by two or more organizations to achieve common goals" (p. 39). They maintained that the nature of the relationship includes "a commitment to: mutual relationships and goals; a jointly developed structure and shared responsibility; mutual authority and accountability for success; and sharing of resources and rewards" (p. 39).

Collaboration connotates a durable and pervasive relationship. Collaboration brings previously separated organizations into a new structure with full commitment to a common mission. Such relationships require comprehensive planning and well defined communication channels operating on many levels. Authority is determined by the collaborative structure. Risk is much greater because each member of the collaboration contributes its own resources and reputation. Resources are pooled or jointly secured and products are shared (Mattessich & Monsey, 1992).

Barbara Gray's (1989) work suggested two major opportunities for collaboration: one related to conflict resolution and another for advancing a shared vision. Collaboration induced by shared visions is intended to advance the collective good of the stakeholders involved. Public and private partnerships developed to address the deteriorating conditions in U.S. cities are illustrative of collaborative efforts across sectors to advance a shared vision.

One can conclude from this discussion that in the human service arena, collaborations are developed to address prevailing social or health problems and a shared vision of how to attack or solve the problems. The shared vision is the glue that binds agencies together in a collaborative venture. A true collaboration is governed by a set of contractual or formal agreements which delineates how authority, interventions, and resources are to be shared by the agencies involved in the collaborative as they seek to solve a specified problem(s).

An Evaluation Framework

Confronted with the lack of a framework for evaluation of collaborative the authors developed an evaluation framework based on a survey of the literature (Harbert, Finnegan, & Reynolds, 1995). The framework is summarized in Figure 1.

Figure 1 suggests that an evaluation of collaboration be approached from a systems perspective which incorporates a conceptual theme that uses interrelated components. The conceptual components are context, process, and outcomes (McLaughlin & Covert, 1984).

The factors which constitute the context dimension influence how the stakeholders will move through the collaborative process and whether or not desired outcomes are achieved (Mattessich & Monsey, 1992). Successful progression through the phases of the collaborative process and completion of process associated tasks determine if outcomes are achieved and the types of outcomes achieved (Flynn & Harbin, 1987; Gray, 1989; Kagan, 1991). The framework also indicates that outcomes of collaborative efforts will differ, depending on the phase of the collaborative process which is being evaluated (Harbert et al., 1995).

The literature suggested that collaboration will not produce successful outcomes unless the context in which it is attempted is conducive to collaboration (Gray, 1989; Mattessich & Monsey, 1992) and the process is skillfully orchestrated (Gray, 1989). Understanding the context in which the collaboration occurs is especially critical in the formative stage of the collaborative process. However, the factors making up the context area need to be reexamined during all phases of the collaboration because they may significantly affect the outcomes of the collaboration during all phases (Gray, 1989; Harbert et al., 1995).

In assessing collaboration, it is necessary to gauge at what point one is entering the process. This can be determined by assessing if the tasks associated with a specific phase have been partially or totally completed. The phases of the collaborative process are developmental and are not totally discrete (Flynn & Harbin, 1987). Consequently, tasks from different phases may occur at the same time, particularly as groups move from one phase to another (Gray, 1989).

In addition to an examination of the context and process, the framework suggests that the outcomes expected of a collaboration will depend on the phase of the collaboration. Outcomes appropriate for collaboration in their formative and developmental phases should focus on the products of collaboration such as common mission, goals and contractual agreement (Baumheier, Welch, & Cook, 1976; Gray, 1989; Kagan, 1991; Magrab, Flynn, & Pelosi, 1985; McLaughlin & Covert, 1984). When collaboration

FIGURE 1

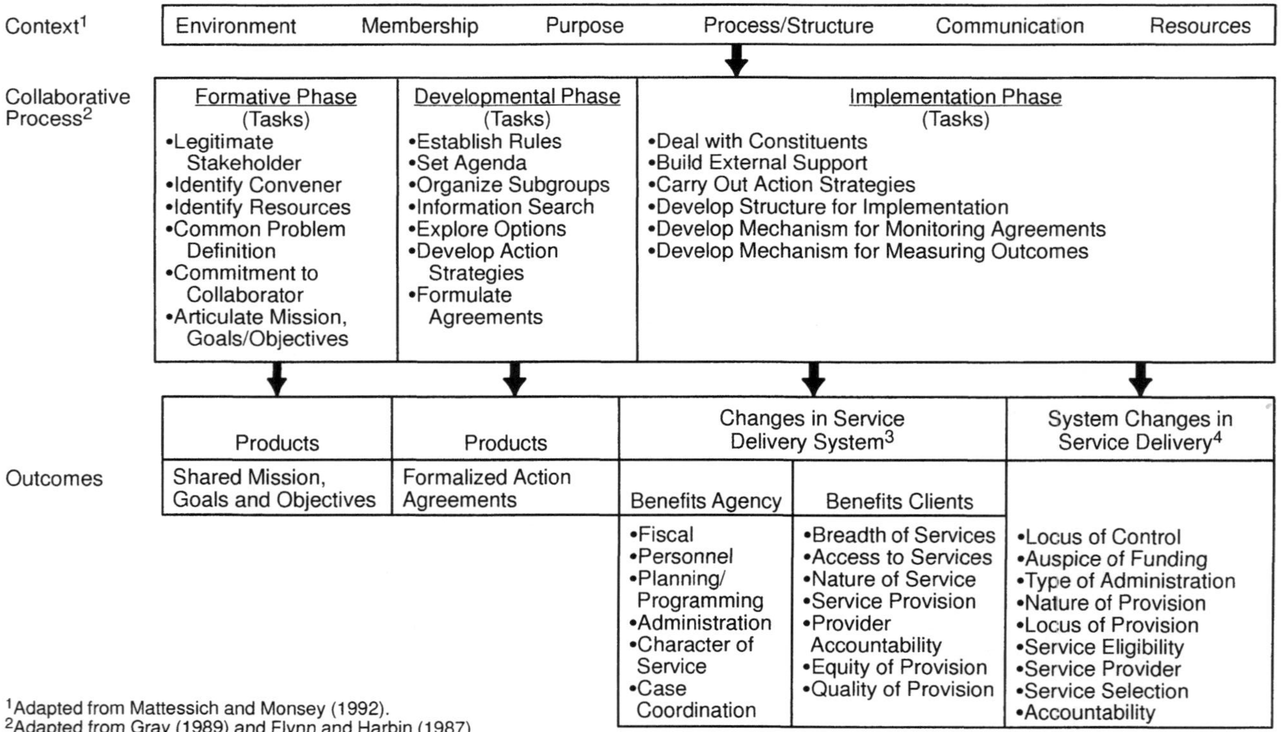

[1]Adapted from Mattessich and Monsey (1992).
[2]Adapted from Gray (1989) and Flynn and Harbin (1987).
[3]Adapted from Baumheier et al. (1976).
[4]Adapted from Gilbert et al. (1993).

has reached the implementation phase, it is appropriate to look for outcomes in terms of changes in the service delivery system or more global systems changes (Baumheier et al., 1976; Kagan, 1991; Magrab et al., 1985; McLaughlin, 1984; Melaville & Blank, 1991).

The framework assumes a comprehensive approach to evaluation that looks at all three components of the framework. It also assumes a longitudinal approach. However, very often those desiring to study interagency collaboration do not become involved in evaluation at the beginning of the collaboration. It is key for the researchers to assess where they are tapping into the collaborative process, whether in the formative, developmental or implementation phase of the process, and to design the study based on the phase.

RESEARCH METHOD

This study was designed as an exploratory case study and, since a definitive analytical framework for conducting this type of study did not exist, the researchers used the framework they developed to design the study. The initial focus of the study was the formative phase of the Children's Initiative collaborative effort. The study took place over an 11-month time period. As suggested by several authors, the phases of the collaborative process are not concrete and may overlap, particularly as groups are moving from one phase to another. This fact was considered as part of the design.

Research Question

The purpose of this exploratory case study was to answer the question, "What factors facilitate or inhibit the interagency collaborative efforts of the Strategic Action Committee to develop a strategic action plan for implementation of a Children's Initiative?"

Sample

A purposive sample was used for this study. It consists of the members of the Children's Initiative Strategic Action Committee (SAC). The Strategic Action Committee is composed of representatives from four key fields of social service provision, Health, Education, Safety and Economic Security, as well as members at large. A total of 28 agencies and organizations are represented on the SAC. The chief executive officer and next highest level administrator of each of the agencies and organizations served as members of the SAC.

Table 1 contains the demographic characteristics of the sample. Time 1 administration included a sample of 33 individuals; of these 60.6% were Chief Executive Officers (CEO). The educational level of the respondents in that group was 30.3% with BA/BS degrees, 33.3% with MA/MS degrees, and 36.4% with PhD/MD/JD degrees. The predominate auspices of the respondents were public nonprofits at 63.6%, the representations of private nonprofits were 30.3%, and 6.1% were from private for profit organizations. The gender of the group was predominately male at 63.6%.

TABLE 1. Demographic Characteristics of the Survey Respondents

	% Baseline Time 1 June, 1994 (N = 33)	% Time 2 May, 1995 (N = 31)
Position		
CEO	60.6	61.3
Education		
BA/BS	30.3	25.8
MA/MS	33.3	35.5
PhD/MD/JD	36.4	38.7
Auspices		
Private nonprofit	30.3	25.8
Public nonprofit	63.6	74.2
Private for profit	6.1	--
Gender–male	63.6	61.3
Age		
20-34	6.3	6.5
35-49	46.9	35.5
50-64	46.9	54.8
65-80	--	35.5
Time in position (years)	Mean = 3.9 (4.0 sd)	Mean = 4.2 (4.2 sd)
Time in organization (years)	Mean = 11.8 (9.5 sd)	Mean = 11.8 (9.5 sd)
Time in profession (years)	Mean = 20.2 (6.0 sd)	Mean = 21.5 (9.0 sd)

The age distribution of the respondents was highest in the 35 to 64 age groups, and those 35-49 and 50-64 both represented 46.9% of the sample. The mean length of time in the respondent's current position was 3.9 years, the mean length of time with their current agency/organization was 11.8 years, and the mean length of time in their chosen profession was 20.2 years.

Comparisons between the respondents at Time 1 and Time 2 did not reveal any statistically significant difference among demographic characteristics.

Data Collection

The framework was used as a guide for the type of data to be collected and analyzed. Data related to the context were collected via a questionnaire distributed to the sample described above. Data related to the collaborative process and outcomes components identified in the framework were based on minutes, drafts, and final reports of the SAC.

Instruments

A questionnaire was developed to solicit opinions of the collaborative group members regarding the degree to which the factors associated with the context were operating. Using a 5-point Likert scale, 50 questions were constructed to explore the context for collaboration suggested by Mattessich and Monsey (1992) and displayed in Figure 1.

The questionnaire was administered for the first time early in the SAC's development, i.e., 5 months after they began meeting. At that time SAC consisted of 37 members representing 28 organizations. Questionnaires were completed by 33 members, representing an 80% response rate.

The questionnaire was administered the second time 11 months later. By this time the membership of SAC had increased to 52. Thirty-one members completed the questionnaire at the second administration, which represents a 60% response rate.

The second type of data collected for the study related to the process and outcomes dimension of the collaborative efforts of the Strategic Action Committee. Documents produced by the Committee, such as minutes, subcommittee report, work plan report, preliminary and final drafts of statements of goals, objectives and strategies, and action plans were systematically reviewed to obtain information on the completion of process tasks and the outcomes of the SAC's efforts over the 11-month period of the study. A form utilizing the categories of delivery system changes suggested by Baumheier (1976) was used to collect and codify information on the outcomes of the SAC's effort.

FINDINGS

Context

The results of the survey of the SAC members examining the context in which the collaboration is occurring are presented using the six broad areas considered important to successful collaborations: environmental, membership, process and structure, communication, purpose, and resources.

The items in the survey used a 5-point Likert-type scale for responses. Responses were strongly disagree, disagree, uncertain, agree, and strongly agree. For ease of presentation responses of agree and strongly agree were combined, and the percentage of all respondents who indicated agreement was calculated. A summary of the results are shown in Table 2 which identifies the number of items related to each factor and the number of items for which there was a consensus among the respondents. Consensus was operationally defined as at least 70% of the respondents agreeing or strongly agreeing with the item.

The environmental area was divided into three areas: a history of previous collaboration (two items), a leadership role in the community (two items), and a favorable political/social environment (four items). The results indicate a consensus that two of the three environmental factors are present. The group members report a history of collaboration and consider themselves to be leaders in the community. There is less agreement, however, about the political/social climate. Of the four items related to this aspect of the environment, a consensus was evident for only one of the items.

Membership is the second general area in which factors associated with favorable collaborations have been identified. Four factors related to membership are considered: mutual respect, understanding and trust (six items); appropriate representation of a cross-section of members of relevant organizations (two items); a perception among members that collaboration is in their self-interest (two items); and an ability of the members to compromise (two items).

A consensus among the respondents reflecting mutual respect, understanding, and trust did not emerge. Consensus was evident for only one of the six items related to this factor. Nor was consensus evident on the two items addressing the representation of SAC. However, the respondents

TABLE 2. Number of Items Where Respondents Reported Consensus with Items Related to Context in Which Collaboration Occurs*

	Number** of items	Time 1*** consensus	Time 2*** consensus
Environmental factors			
1. Previous history of collaboration	2	2	2
2. Leadership role in community	2	2	2
3. Favorable political/social climate	4	1	1
Membership characteristics			
1. Mutual respect, understanding, and trust	6	1	1
2. Appropriate cross-section of members	2	0	0
3. Members see collaboration as in their self-interest	2	2	2
4. Ability to compromise	2	0	2
Process/structure			
1. Members share a stake in process/outcome	5	2	4
2. Multiple layers of decision-makers involved	4	1	1
3. Development of clear roles/policy guidelines	1	1	1
4. Adaptability of collaborative group	3	2	2
Communication			
1. Open and frequent communication	4	1	3
2. Establish informal/formal communication links	4	2	3
Purpose			
1. Concrete attainable goals and objectives	3	0	3
2. Shared vision	2	0	2
3. Unique purpose	1	0	0
Resources			
1. Skilled convener	4	3	3
2. Sufficient funds	1	0	0

* 70% or more of respondents agreed or strongly agreed.
** Total number of questions for each factor.
*** Time 1, June 1994; Time 2, May 1995.

generally agreed that participation in the collaborative effort represented by the SAC is in their own self-interest. Additionally, at the second administration of the survey the ability of the members of SAC to compromise was recognized.

The next general area examined in the survey addressed the process/structure of the collaborative group. This area is subdivided into four factors: members share a stake in both process and outcome (five items); multiple layers of decision making (four items); development of clear roles and policy guidelines (one item); and adaptability (three items).

In this area the number of items of consensus rose from two to four between Time 1 and Time 2 for the factor reflecting the members' stake in the process/outcome. There is less consensus about the involvement of multiple layers of decision making in the collaboration. Consensus was reached on only one of the four items examining this aspect of the SAC actions. Consensus was reached on two of the three items related to adaptability. In this area there was no consensus that the SAC is structured to sustain itself in the midst of major change.

The fourth area impacting on successful collaboration relates to the level of communication among the members of the collaboration. Two factors of communications were addressed by the items in the survey: the openness and frequency of communication (four items), and the nature of informal and formal communications links (four items). Over the course of the two administrations of this survey, the respondents reported improvements in the communication patterns of the members of SAC. For both of the factors of communication examined, consensus was evident at the second administration of the survey for three of the four items addressing the factor.

Purpose was the fifth area associated with successful collaborations examined. Concrete attainable goals and objectives (three items), a shared vision (two items), and a unique purpose (one item) are all factors of this area that tend to relate to successful collaborations. The results of these items in the survey clearly show that the SAC members have tended to modify their views about the purpose of the SAC over time. By the second administration, consensus was achieved for all of the items related to this area with the exception of the item related to the unique purpose of the collaboration.

The final area related to successful collaborations examined in the survey concerns the resources available to the collaborative effort. In particular, a skilled convener and sufficient funds are considered essential. For this collaboration, there appeared to be a general agreement that the convener was skilled. However, consensus was not indicated about the adequacy of the resources available for the collaborative effort.

Collaborative Process

An effort was made to determine where the collaborative group was in the process over the 11-month time period of this study. This was done by determining if specific process tasks were completed for specific phases of the collaboration. Table 3 identifies the tasks completed.

TABLE 3. Collaborative Process Tasks Completed

	Tasks Completed
Formative Phase:	
Identification of stakeholders	X
Legitimation of stakeholders	X
Identification of convener	X
Identification of resources to carry out the collaboration	X
Common definition of the problem	X
Articulation of mission	X
Articulation of goals	X
Articulation of objectives	
Developmental Phase:	
Establish ground rules	
Set the agenda	
Organize subgroups	X
Search for information	X
Explore options	
Develop action strategies	
Reach formal or informal agreements as to what each stakeholder will do/or contribute	
Implementation Phase	
Deal with constituents	X
Build external support	X
Carry out action strategies	
Develop a structure for implementation	
Develop mechanisms for monitoring agreements	
Develop mechanisms for measurement of outcomes	

Most of the tasks associated with the formative phase of the collaborative process were completed during the study period. Stakeholders were identified, legitimated, and engaged; a convener was identified and engaged; resources were identified, accessed, and a staff hired to support the group; the group arrived at a common definition of the problem; and the SAC members made a commitment to collaborations relative to a solution to the problem. The members also articulated and agreed on a common mission and goals. They did not, however, articulate a specific set of objectives as to how the goals would be achieved. During the study period, SAC began to move into some of the tasks associated with the developmental phase such as organizing subgroups and joint information searches.

They also became involved with tasks associated with the implementation phase such as dealing with constituents and building external support.

Outcomes of the SAC's Collaborative Effort

An assessment of the outcomes of the efforts of the SAC showed that expected outcomes related to the formative phase of the collaborative process were produced. They adopted a shared vision, mission, and goals. The vision and mission of the Children's Initiative was prescribed for the SAC by the Initiative Steering Committee. The vision was to create a more nurturing and supportive community of people and organizations that places top priority on children and families and encourages them to reach their potential. The mission is to strengthen children and families by working for integrated service delivery systems that promote the values of collaboration, prevention, and measurable outcomes in the fields of health, education, safety, and economic security.

One of the first goals of the SAC, to adopt the prescribed mission and vision, occurred early in the group's deliberations. It took almost a year, however, for the group to decide on a set of goals aimed at achieving the Initiative's mission and vision. At the time this study was completed, they had neither agreed upon specific objectives for achieving these goals nor were formal agreements arrived at for achievement of goals and objectives.

In an effort to operationalize the vision of the Children's Initiative, the SAC developed a two-pronged approach by articulating two sets of goals: one set identified as program goals and another identified as systems change strategies. Four program goals focus areas were identified: children ages 0 to 6 years of age (Zero to Six); providing a safe and nonviolent environment for children and youth (Safety and Violence); assisting youth make the transition from school to career (School to Career); and creating families and neighborhood supports to meet the needs of children (Community and Family Development). Goals and subgoals were articulated for each of the focus areas. The goals and the number of subgoals for each are identified below.

Within the Zero to Six focus area, three goals were identified: infants will be born healthy (three subgoals); children will stay healthy (six subgoals); and children will start school ready to learn (five subgoals). In the Safety and Violence focus area, three goals were articulated: children and youth will experience an increase in peace through a reduction of intentional violence (six subgoals); children and youth will experience an increase in safety through a reduction of unintentional injury and death (four subgoals); and children will be protected and nurtured through a reduction in abuse and neglect (four subgoals). The School to Career focus included two goals: youth will be prepared to enter the world of work and/or pursue post-secondary education (five subgoals); and youth will experience an increase in the number of high skilled, high wage jobs through the enhancement of economic development (four subgoals). The Community and Family Development focus includes two goals: increase family effectiveness (five subgoals); and increase neighborhood effectiveness (three subgoals). In total the SAC identified 10 major program goals with 45 subgoals.

Seven system change strategies were identified with 18 subgoals. The strategies included: operational effectiveness (three subgoals); youth partnership (two subgoals); collaborative grant seeking (one subgoal); data integration (one subgoal); results based children's budget (three subgoals); public policy council (one goal); and community engagement (three subgoals). Each goal/strategy statement and its corresponding subgoals were analyzed to determine if they would lead to specific operational objectives that would effect changes in service delivery systems or more global system changes.

Table 4 shows that of the 45 program subgoals, approximately 30 were related to potential changes in the service delivery system as related to agencies and clients; one related to system change. The 15 program subgoals that did not fall into the service delivery system change category were directed to realms outside the service delivery systems such as the media, businesses, neighborhoods, families, and individual behaviors.

The system strategies were conceived to be system change strategies but with the possible exception of one, these strategies did not fit the definition of system change outcomes suggested by Melaville and Blank (1991). They maintained that collaborative efforts aimed at systems change are empowered authoritatively either by collective "clout" or legally by the state or other entities to call for new directions in systemwide programming and make the budgetary revisions and administrative changes necessary to implement them.

The language contained in some of these systems strategies were more reflective of possible outcomes related to changes in the service delivery system. Of the 18 strategy subgoals, eight were directed to changes in the service delivery system. The others were related to areas outside of the social service arena. These are illustrated in Table 4.

The system strategy that had the most potential for a systems change outcome was public policy. This strategy contains language related to a commitment to collective advocacy in an effort to influence governmental policy decisions related to programs for children and families. Two strategies, youth partnership and community engagement, were directed at realms

TABLE 4. Outcomes of Collaboration

Implementation phase (projected)	# Program subgoals	# System strategies
Changes in the service delivery system of benefit to agencies		
Fiscal-shared, redistribution of resources		2
Personnel–joint use of staff, reassignment	6	3
Planning and programming–joint planning, collaborative programming	5	1
Administration–joint effort, restructured	4	2
Character of client consumer services–redefined, collaborative delivery		
Client or case coordination–team approach, interagency case management	2	
Changes in the service delivery system of benefit to client		
Breadth of service, delivery system–comprehensive, categorical, constricted		
Access to service–single access, multiple access	1	
Nature of service system–comprehensive, coordinated, fragmented services	9	
Service provision–agency basis, contractual voucher		
Provider accountability–to funder or to the client/consumer		
Equity in provision–common standards of provision, differential standards of provision	1	
Quality of provision–consistency, continuity, efficiency	2	
System changes in delivery system		
Auspices of funding–single source, multiple source		
Type of administration–centralized, decentralized		
Nature of provision–monetary, in-kind, preventive, developmental, remedial	1	
Locus of provision–single provider, multiple provider		
Service eligibility–universality, selectivity		
Service selection–expert's choice, client/consumer's choice		
Accountability–based on numbers served and results		
TOTAL	31	8

outside the service delivery system and did not fit any of the categories of service delivery collaborative outcomes identified in the study.

DISCUSSION

The Strategic Action Committee (SAC) in the time period under study was able to achieve most of the types of outcomes expected in the formative phase of interagency collaborative efforts. They were able to articulate a shared vision, mission, and goals. Although the SAC articulated goals that are reflective of the vision and mission of the Initiative, the number of goals established for the Children's Initiative raise serious questions regarding whether they all can be attained, particularly in the context of collaborative interagency efforts. In other cities attempting similar but more modest approaches to effect system changes for children and youth through collaboration, a number of difficulties have been suggested. The Annie E. Casey Foundation has funded five cities in the United States to form collaboratives to address three major goals related to problems of disadvantaged urban youths. A report of the Foundation suggests that attainment of collaborative action around only three goals is difficult, complex, time consuming, and fraught with many obstacles.

Moreover, although the mission of the Children's Initiative is focused on strengthening children and families by working for integrated service delivery systems that permit the values of collaboration, prevention, and measurable outcomes, the findings suggest that a number of the goals and systems change strategies adopted for the Initiative are much broader and more comprehensive than is suggested by the mission. A number of the goals and strategies adopted for the Initiative suggest an intent to influence areas beyond the service delivery systems such as the media, business, neighborhoods, communities, and individual behaviors. By enumerating so many goals and expanding the arenas to be influenced through collaborative actions, it would appear an already difficult and highly complex effort is made even more complex and challenging. Here again, the Casey Foundation experience suggests that perhaps containment of the number of goals to be achieved and arenas to be affected in a collaborative effort may be a more prudent approach for actual goals attainment.

After 18 months of effort the group still appeared to be in the formative phase. They were unable to move to the point of articulating a set of specific objectives for achieving agreed upon goals which would then allow the SAC to move solidly into the developmental phase. A number of tasks associated with the development phase relate to the operationalization of objectives and the establishment of an action plan to carry out these objectives. Without these objectives the tasks associated with the developmental phase cannot be completed. The Children's Initiative will not become a true collaboration until the developmental phase of the collaborative process is completed. The types of goals established for the Children's Initiative, with the possible exception of one or two, appear to be propelling the group to outcomes related to changes in the service delivery system.

The survey of the SAC members suggested that for the most part the context dimension which includes the factors associated with successful collaborations were operating for the group. The environment appeared to be conducive to the group's efforts. The group was not at a high level of consensus about the membership characteristics of the SAC, although they were in strong agreement about the group seeing collaboration in their own self-interest. There was neither a high level of agreement among the members about the extent of mutual respect, understanding, and trust among the organizations involved, nor whether all appropriate groups representing children were involved. With respect to the process/structure factor, the group was in strong agreement that they shared a stake in the process and outcomes of the collaborative effort. However, they were not in agreement regarding the efforts of the members to include and inform lower level administrative personnel of their organization about the activities or proposed actions of the SAC. In addition, over time there was a decrease in the level of agreement among members regarding whether structure/process was adaptable and would allow needed changes to occur.

It would appear from the results that the level of communication within and among the members improved over time. There was also a dramatic change in the members' perception of the purpose of the SAC effort. Members' opinions regarding the ability of the group to develop a shared vision and concrete, attainable goals and objectives improved over time. There was a slight drop, however, in the perception of the SAC members with regard to the uniqueness of the mission and goals of the Children's Initiative compared to those of their own organizations. There was strong agreement relative to resources on the skill of the SAC convener but not a high level of agreement as to the adequacy of resources to support the SAC's efforts.

Within the context dimensions, there may be difficulties in two factor areas, membership and process/structure. This perhaps explains why the SAC is not moving more expeditiously into the developmental and implementation phases of the collaborative process. The results of the survey suggest there is not a high level of mutual respect, understanding, and trust among group members. Gray (1989) indicated that there is a perceived risk involved in entering collaborative endeavors because the process is unfamiliar and the outcomes uncertain. Mattessich and Monsey (1992) maintained that the risk is greater in collaborative arrangements than in other types of interagency efforts. In a collaboration members contribute their resources and reputations. Without a high level of mutual respect, understanding, and trust, it is highly unlikely that members of a collaborative will move easily into the development phases of the collaborative process. It is in the development phase that they develop formalized agreements in which authority, resources, and reputation are surrendered to a true collaborative effort.

Another factor in the member category that may explain why it is taking longer than expected for the SAC to move to the next phase of the collaborative process has to do with the composition of the group and perhaps its size. Rist et al. (1980), in a study of collaborations among education and employment/training organizations, found that the greater the number of organizations involved, the greater the complexity of the linkage system and the amount of time invested in maintaining these linkages. The study suggested that there is a point of diminishing returns for projects as they link themselves to other organizations and agencies. They also suggested that in such complex collaboratives it was found that overextension of senior staff has a direct impact upon the lengthy time lag that many projects experienced in becoming operational. In addition, with complexity of linkages, the number of decisions to be made and the number of participants involved means an increasing accumulation of delays in implementation. At the beginning of this study the SAC included representation from approximately 16 agencies and organizations. At the time the study was completed, there were approximately 28 agencies and organizations involved with the SAC. The lack of trust, understanding, and respect among the members and the complexity of the SAC's membership and its size may be impeding its progress in the collaborative process and its ability to move forward to formalization of a true collaboration effort for the Children's Initiative.

The other factor which may explain why the group has not moved to the next phase is a change in perception in the process/structure domain. It appears that members, after 18 months into the collaborative process, no longer feel as strongly that the process and structure are flexible enough to allow needed changes to occur. Over time the group appears to have less confidence that mechanisms are in place to monitor the progress of the group and to make needed changes in process or structure, goals, membership, decision-making structure, and so forth. This change in attitude on the part of the SAC members may suggest that the group is at a juncture when such changes are needed to move forward in a productive manner.

Opinions of the SAC members relative to the membership and process/structure factors may be interrelated. Perhaps given the complexity of composition and size of the group, a different process and structure than the one currently in place is needed to facilitate the group's efforts.

CONCLUSIONS

Children have been identified as an at-risk group in this country, and efforts are underway in many sectors to correct this condition. In times of shrinking resources collaboration is being promoted as a better means of meeting the needs of children and families. A Children's Initiative collaborative was developed in a large metropolitan area to address the problems of children and an effort was made to study this collaborative venture. The study tapped into this collaborative effort in the formative phase and focused on those dimensions that influenced and facilitated the efforts of the Strategic Action Committee of the Children's Initiative to develop a strategic action plan to implement the goals of the Initiative. The study design tested an evaluation framework developed by the researchers.

The results of the study suggest that after approximately 18 months of deliberation the Strategic Action Committee of the Children's Initiative have successfully completed most of the outcomes associated with the formative phase of the collaborative process. They have agreed upon a shared vision, mission, and goals. Although goals have been identified for the Initiative, the large number identified and the breadth of the goals, some of which go beyond the parameters of social services delivery system, raise questions about the reality of attaining them all.

Moreover, the Strategic Action Committee was not successful during the period of the study to achieve one outcome related to this phase, the delineating of a set of objectives for carrying out the agreed upon goal. Development of a set of operational objectives for achieving the Initiative goals will allow the SAC to move solidly into the developmental phase of the collaborative process. Unless the SAC moves into this phase and successfully completes the tasks associated with it, they will neither develop into a true collaboration nor will they be able to move into the implementation phase of the collaborative process and achieve its goals. The results also suggest that two factors may be impeding the progress of the SAC, one related to the membership of the group and the other related to the process and structure under which the group operates.

This study focused on the formative phase of the SAC's collaborative efforts. The framework used for the study assumes a systemic, longitudinal approach to evaluation of collaboration. Given that it takes several years for a collaborative to implement and achieve its objectives, it would be necessary to continue the study of the Children's Initiative into the developmental and implementation phases to access the outcomes of the Initiative. A study of the developmental phase would assess if the SAC develops a set of operational objectives that enables the creation of a strategic action plan and formal agreements for carrying out the plan. A study of the implementation phase would focus on successful implementation of the strategic action plan and the types of outcomes achieved.

Given the findings of this study, several questions surfaced related to interagency collaborative efforts which may warrant further study. For example, is there an optimal number of agencies and organizations that can successfully engage collectively in a collaborative endeavor to assure a positive outcome for the collaborative? Is it advisable for collaboratives to focus on a few high priority goals and objectives to assure attainment of a few goals rather than to enumerate a broad set of comprehensive goals for which attainment of all might be less likely? Another question that requires review is: How within the collaborative context can a level of trust be established among the stakeholders which will enable them to surrender control of authority and resources to the collaborative effort?

There are a few issues for consideration which can be gleaned from the study that may be of use to social agency administrators who plan to be engaged or are engaged in interagency collaboration. When administrators of social agencies are asked to become involved in a collaborative endeavor to achieve a shared vision, they should be aware that they are engaging in a venture that is very time consuming and may require several years of commitment. In addition, the more organizations that are involved in the collaboration, the greater will be the time commitment required to maintain interagency collaborative relationships. Moreover, if the interagency effort results in a true collaboration, administrators need to be prepared and willing to relinquish control of certain resources and decision-making authority to the collaborative effort. Finally, because collaboration requires long-term commitments, the nature and character of the collaborative effort may change over time and the stakeholders need to be assured that the governing structure of the collaborative is flexible enough to allow these changes to occur and that mechanisms are in place to assure that they occur smoothly without disrupting the collaborative.

REFERENCES

Alaszewski, A., & Harrison, L. (1988). Literature review: Collaboration and coordination between welfare agencies. *British Journal of Social Work, 18*, 635-647.

Annie E. Casey Foundation. (1995). *The path of most resistance: Reflections on lessons learned from new futures*. Baltimore, MD: The Annie E. Casey Foundation.

Baumheier, E.C., Welch, H.H., & Cook, C.C. (1976). *Interagency linkages in vocational rehabilitation*. Denver: University of Denver, Regional Rehabilitation Research Institute, Center for Social Research and Development.

Children's Defense Fund. (1992). *The state of American children*. Washington, DC: Children's Defense Fund.

Edelman, M.W. (1987). *Families in peril: An agenda for social change*. Cambridge, MA: Harvard University Press.

Flynn, C.C., & Harbin, G.L. (1987). Evaluating interagency coordination efforts using a multidimensional, interactional, developmental paradigm. *Remedial and Special Education*, *8*(3), 35-44.

Gage, R.W. (1976). Integration of human services delivery systems. *Public Welfare*, *34*(1), 27-33.

Gray, B. (1989). *Collaborating: Finding common ground for multiplier problems*. San Francisco: Jossey-Bass.

Grubb, N., & Lazerson, M. (1983). *Broken promises: How America fails its children*. New York: Basic Books.

Guthrie, G.P., & Guthrie, L.F. (1991, Winter). Streamlining interagency collaboration for youth at risk. *Educational Leadership*, 17-22.

Harbert, A.S., Finnegan, D., & Reynolds, B. (1995). *A framework for evaluating interagency collaboration*. Unpublished manuscript: San Diego State University.

Kagan, S.L. (1991). *United we stand: Collaboration for child care and early education services*. New York: Teachers College Press.

Kammerman, S. (1989). Toward a child policy decade. *Child Welfare*, *68*(4), 371-390.

Magrab, P., Flynn, C., & Pelosi, J. (1985). *Assessing interagency coordination through process evaluation*. Chapel Hill: North Carolina University, Frank Porter Graham Center, State Technical Assistance Resource Team. (ERIC Document Reproduction Service No. ED 266 581.)

Mattessich, P.W., & Monsey, B.R. (1992). *Collaboration: What makes it work*? St. Paul, MN: Amherst Wilder Foundation.

McLaughlin, J.A., & Covert, R.C. (1984). *Evaluating interagency partnerships to connect children and families with comprehensive services*. Chapel Hill: North Carolina University, State Technical Assistance Resource Team. (ERIC Document Reproduction Service No. ED 255 022.)

Melaville, A., & Blank, M. (1991). *What it takes: Structuring interagency partnerships to connect children and families with comprehensive services*. Washington, DC: Education and Human Services Consortium.

Rein, M. (1970). *Social policy*. New York: Random House.

Rist, R.C. et al. (1980). *Patterns of collaboration: The CETA/school linkage, An analysis of inter-institutional linkages between education and employment/training organizations*. (Interim Report #4.) Ithaca, NY: Cornell University,

Youthwork National Policy Study. (ERIC Document Reproductive Service No. ED 224 901.)
Scales, P., & Brunk, B. (1990). Keeping children on top of the states agenda. *Child Welfare, 71*(8), 500-503.
Schorr, L. (1988). *Within our reach.* New York: Anchor Press.
Sidel, R. (1986). *Women and children last.* New York: Viking.
Steiner, G. (1981). *The futility of family policy.* Washington, DC: The Brookings Institute.
Swan, W.W., & Morgan, J.L. (1991). *Collaborating for comprehensive services for young children and their families: The local interagency coordinating council.* Baltimore, MD: Paul H. Brookes.
Zald, M.N. (1969). The structure of society and social service integration. *Social Science Quarterly, 50*, 557-567.
Zimmerman, S.S. (1988). *Understanding family policy.* Newbury Park, CA: Sage.

Launching a Family-Centered, Neighborhood-Based Human Services System: Lessons from Working the Hallways and Street Corners

Katherine L. Armstrong, DPH

SUMMARY. The author describes Contra Costa County's efforts to implement Healthy Families 2000, the County's vision of neighborhood-based, family-centered, comprehensive integrated services in two of the county's unincorporated areas, North Richmond and Bay Point. Contra Costa County is one of six bay area counties, northeast of San Francisco. It has nearly 800,000 residents and is home to some of the wealthiest communities in the state as well as some of the poorest neighborhoods. This article provides a systematic review of the process and a discussion of the operating practices and principles guiding Contra Costa's significant effort to change its service delivery approach, anticipating that this experience might be helpful to others as they develop a neighborhood-based human services partnership with community leaders and residents. *[Article copies available for a fee from The Haworth Document Delivery Service: 1-800-342-9678. E-mail address: getinfo@haworth.com]*

Katherine L. Armstrong is Executive Director, Zellerback Family Fund, 120 Montgomery Street, Suite 2125, San Francisco, CA 94104.

[Haworth co-indexing entry note]: "Launching a Family-Centered, Neighborhood-Based Human Services System: Lessons from Working the Hallways and Street Corners." Armstrong, Katherine L. Co-published simultaneously in *Administration in Social Work* (The Haworth Press, Inc.) Vol. 21, No. 3/4, 1997, pp. 109-126; and: *Human Services Integration* (ed: Michael J. Austin) The Haworth Press, Inc., 1997, pp. 109-126. Single or multiple copies of this article are available for a fee from The Haworth Document Delivery Service [1-800-342-9678, 9:00 a.m. - 5:00 p.m. (EST). E-mail address: getinfo@haworth.com].

THE PROCESS OF ORGANIZATIONAL AND COMMUNITY CHANGE

Nearly five years ago, Contra Costa County began its long journey toward the development of neighborhood-based, family-centered services when its Board of Supervisors and the Youth Services Board (YSB), a policy making body made up of the Directors of Social Service, Probation, Health, Community Services, and the County Executive, Superintendent County of Schools, Juvenile Court Judge and children's advocates, made a commitment to translating the county's successful Inter-Agency Family Preservation Program into system-wide change. The county's access with Family Preservation taught a number of valuable lessons. Through an inter-agency commitment to families it had prevented out-of-home placements, reduced foster care costs, and helped improve the family life of participants. The county now had tangible evidence that concentrating on the entire family, engaging families as active partners, and assisting families within the context of the community resulted in better functioning families and cost savings. Just as significant as these improvements, the county had learned that Social Services, Health Services, Probation, and Community Services could work together successfully when presented with a common goal, a unified structure for delivering services, and a mandated reporting of results.

Much of the success of this undertaking can be attributed to the fact that both the Board of Supervisors and the Youth Services Board were committed to creating a human services system that was community-based, family-centered, comprehensive, and involved inter-agency collaboration. All involved were committed to improving the well-being of the county's children and their families and preventing the costly family crises which now absorbed most of the county's resources and attention.

A consultant was hired for a three-year period to assist the YSB realize this goal of strengthening families. During the next three-and-a-half years the consultant:

- drafted the vision statement and strategic plan, obtained feedback, made necessary improvements, and communicated the vision to every significant group in the county;
- staffed and directed the work of the YSB and its newly created inter-agency managerial planning body, the Service Integration Management Team (SIMT), in carrying out the day-to-day work of designing and implementing community-based service integration;
- completed the analysis needed to select the key neighborhoods for development;

- engaged and motivated neighborhood residents, leaders, and community agencies in the two communities selected for piloting the new system of services;
- participated in extensive negotiations with unions, agency staff, and community-based organizations;
- helped develop the programmatic and physical infrastructure for relocating inter-agency, integrated services into the neighborhoods;
- consulted on the development of a proposal to become an AB-1741 service integration pilot county, the state's fast track for state waivers; and
- assisted with training and staff development issues.

Developing a Vision and Strategic Plan

The YSB faced the daunting challenge of determining how to decentralize county-wide services into a neighborhood-based service delivery system while confined within a rigid web of state and Federal regulations and categorical funding. In addition, YSB members were preoccupied with making severe budget cuts. In this environment, it was important to carve out a change process that allowed for risk-taking, and gave staff time to learn from mistakes, but also imposed as little disruption as possible on the entire human service system.

The first step was to create a unified vision, agree on a set of operating principles and draft a strategic plan. This process took a year and entailed intensive communication and collaboration with staff at many levels within each of the County Departments of Social Services, Health, Probation, Community Services, and the Juvenile Court, the schools, community groups, and children's advocates.

YSB members soon agreed that the development of neighborhood-based, family-centered, integrated services should be targeted to those communities with the highest number of residents living in poverty, and to neighborhoods in which there lived a significant number of clients known to three or more departments or receiving at least four different services. Members decided to pilot this new approach in the identified high risk neighborhoods that also had community leaders receptive and willing to form partnerships with the county.

The process for targeting communities included a data match of the client files from Social Services, Health Services and Probation. Through a geographical mapping of the data match findings, the YSB identified nine neighborhoods where service utilization was greatest, where there lived a large number of families using four or more services of the departments of Social Services (Child Welfare and Income Maintenance) Health, and Probation. High on the list of the nine eligible communities were the county's unincorporated areas of North Richmond and Bay Point/West Pittsburgh. The population characteristics of these unincorporated areas reflected many high risk factors (for example, 50% of residents have not graduated from high school, 34% are unemployed, a high number of children are in kinship foster care, the immunization rate is lower than average, and the infant mortality and morbidity rates are higher than average).

Fortuitously, at the same time the Board of Supervisors and the YSB were completing the strategic plan and finishing up the analysis of the county's service utilization, both North Richmond and Bay Point community members were beginning to organize. Leaders from these communities had recently approached the Board of Supervisors demanding changes in the way all services (including police, transportation, and employment) were delivered to their residents. This new pressure on the board to dramatically change the way services were provided to these two neighborhoods influenced the YSB to choose North Richmond and Bay Point for its first two pilot service integration centers.

Learning About the Neighborhoods and Engaging Residents

One of the key operating principles guiding the service integration effort was a commitment to design the neighborhood services system to meet the needs of families and residents. This required an extensive needs assessment of the communities and establishing new opportunities to hear from clients and residents about what they needed and wanted. The vehicle chosen for this endeavor was to join with the local schools to apply for a California State Department Healthy Start planning grant. The Healthy Start Program, begun in 1991, provides funding to schools with a large percentage of students living in poverty to work partnership with parents, county, city and community based organizations to improve the health and educational performance of their students. With funding obtained via Healthy Start, both North Richmond and Bay Point conducted focus groups, interviews, and town meetings, and completed a resource mapping of the available services, programs, and strengths in the community. The Healthy Start planning process brought many people to the table for the first time and started the dialogue among parents, community-based organizations, schools, and county services about community needs.

During the next year, as the Healthy Start planning effort was under way, North Richmond residents successfully advocated for the creation of a local governance structure, the Municipal Advisory Council (MAC), that reported directly to the Board of Supervisors. Community leaders now had a means to advocate for more access to and accountability from the Board about how county services were delivered in their neighborhood. The North Richmond MAC developed its own strategic plan, incorporating the results from the Healthy Start needs assessment as well as findings from their systematic review of county-delivered services in the community. The North Richmond MAC leadership worked closely with the consultant and county staff guiding the process of county service integration for the North Richmond community. With support from the Zellerbach Family Fund, the MAC was able to fund their own priority projects and hire local people to deliver the programs. In the Bay Point community, a MAC had been authorized during the previous year and a MAC council member was involved with the Healthy Start needs assessment planning process and service integration planning and implementation.

YSB's motivation to improve local access to services and the new grassroots pressure placed on the Board of Supervisors created the needed tension and catalyst to spark dialogue ensured that the system changes were responsive to clients and families who lived in the neighborhoods. The consultant helped establish a mutually supportive and interactive process that allowed community building efforts to proceed independently, but in relationship to the extensive, internal department-level planning required before any services could actually move from central offices to the neighborhood or shift from categorical services to a family-centered and holistic approach.

Negotiating with Staff

Preparing staff for work in the new neighborhood-based, family-centered, service integration teams had two stages. The first stage involved staff selection and training, including:

- deciding what programs and staff, in what combinations, would be located in the neighborhoods;
- developing new job descriptions and determining how staff would be supervised and managed;
- drafting a training curriculum;
- gaining union support; and
- recruiting and selecting staff.

The second stage began immediately after all staff members had been selected, trained and located in the neighborhood centers. This stage required a reassessment and modification of everything that had been decided and begun during the first stage. A range of unanticipated conflicts emerged when staff were transferred from categorical programs, with no history of working together, into new teams responsible for serving the same clients and community.

Language was a huge problem. Workers used similar words, but the same word often had completely different meanings to the social worker, the eligibility worker, the public health nurse, the probation officer and the substance abuse counselor. It took some time together before the team members realized that they were all using different definitions, and even longer to develop common language and definitions of "family-centered, community-based, comprehensive, inter-agency case management," "community involvement," and "partnerships."

Personnel had difficulty respecting each other's work. Tension ran high between disciplines as they struggled with each other in forming a common approach to clients and their needs. Categorical rules and regulations continued to obstruct team relations and cause daily frustration. Departments found it challenging to cope with members of their own staff who were now functioning very differently from their mainstream workers. Turf issues among service providers remained at the heart of every discussion.

Contra Costa County staff struggled with the notion of self-managed teams because the traditional top-down supervision and control did not fit the demand for flexibility in a decentralized service system. However, the concept of a self-managed team was very troublesome for practically everyone–unions, managers, and staff–and continues to evolve as a new form of practice with more experience and training. The county engaged in extensive union negotiation for at least six months before the teams were recruited and selected, and union negotiations continue to be a key aspect of the implementation process. Union members participate in the SIMT and are among the staff operating in the two neighborhood centers. Five different unions were involved in negotiations about every operational issue and assignment of work tasks. Individual unions had concerns which dealt primarily with their own membership; thus, complying with one union's request sometimes placed management in conflict with another union. Management's responsibility was to help everyone reach some consensus before operations could proceed. Many of the initial discussions revolved around issues of safety, workload, and people working outside of existing job classifications. Together, labor and management worked through the design of the management information system, site selection and renovation, site configuration, job descriptions, confidentiality, training, staff development, and how the self-managed team concept would work.

The multitude of day-to-day frustrations quickly became serious obstacles to changing service delivery, raising many reasons to question the whole concept of neighborhood-based service integration. Commitment had to be constantly articulated and communicated by the Board of Supervisors, the YSB, and the County Administrator to all participants to keep everyone on track and moving through these difficulties. This was a top-down change process, but many at every level wanted the same changes. Throughout the entire process, participants continued to struggle with a simple fact: while most of us are in favor of making improvements, few like to make changes in their own world; almost all of us prefer that someone else do the changing.

Negotiating with the State

At the same time the SIMT was working through the operational issues, a study was completed which documented a list of state and federal waivers needed to blend categorical funding streams and redirect staff time from paperwork into prevention activities. This in-depth analysis of departmental operations documented how clients moved through the programs, from intake through exit, noting non-productive activities and requirements imposed on the departments. The county applied for and obtained AB-1741 status, which allowed five county pilots to receive waivers needed to support service integration.

Negotiating with Community Representatives

There were two key aspects to team members' work with communities. One involved establishing new kinds of relationships with the center's new clients, those who receive direct services from the team members. The other aspect required establishing a positive working relationship between the team and the community as a whole. This meant working with the MACs and with the Healthy Start Program as well as other community groups and representatives. This was a new experience for staff and involved considerable on the job learning and experimentation.

Staff were able to establish new positive relationships with their clients more easily than developing a community-wide perspective necessary to build constructive neighborhood relationships. All client participation in the neighborhood centers was voluntary. Team members had to go door-to-door and persuade clients to transfer their cases from the central office to the neighborhood center. This dramatically changed the relationship between workers and clients and set the stage for the kind of individualized attention clients are now receiving. Because workers had to persuade their clients to join the center, staff members felt very responsible for adapting services to better meet client needs, and they assertively advocated with department management to change rigid policies and procedures that affect client services.

While the county engaged in restructuring, re-configuring and dealing with internal issues, the neighborhood representatives were becoming more organized and began advocating for specific service priorities: jobs, increased public safety, and increased after school recreation. There was ongoing tension between what the community viewed as its primary needs and what the county could actually provide under existing categorical funding until the waivers were approved.

The teams continue to learn how to work with neighborhood leadership. Turf struggles exist in the neighborhoods and it is not always clear who is speaking for whom. It is not uncommon to find significant disagreements among neighborhood groups about what is best for the community. Staff have found that the best methods for adapting to community work involve patience, perseverance and relationship-building.

PRACTICE PRINCIPLES FOR MANAGING ORGANIZATIONAL AND COMMUNITY CHANGE

The management principles that impact leaders in the process of change center on four broad tasks–making a personal commitment, re-defining ourselves and our roles, planning for implementation, and moving from planning to action.

Making a Personal Commitment

Implementing a new vision of human services is time-consuming, tedious, and hard work, but not impossible. It requires a personal investment in converting the existing set of mandated department activities into a transforming vision. There usually is broad consensus about the merit of a family centered, neighborhood-based strategy. However, if one lacks passion and the necessary energy, it is impossible to move through the overwhelming inertia that exists in the public sector or to cope with the multiple roadblocks and barriers faced at every turn. Directors of Departments of Social Services interested in promoting family-centered, neighborhood human services should consider the following soul-searching questions:

- Does the vision of a family-centered, neighborhood human service system truly reflect our own vision of the ideal?

- Do we really believe that this vision, if implemented, will make the difference in the lives of our clients, workers and the community?
- Is this a good time to handle the increased responsibilities associated with the needed changes?
- Are we prepared to deal with the inertia, ingrained practices and the resistance we will uncover as we try to change ourselves and our department's practice?
- Are we willing to devote the necessary attention to managing change while handling the ongoing pressures imposed on us by the state or county?
- Are we willing to invest the effort to learn new habits and competencies related to:

    - re-engineering techniques and entrepreneurial approaches;
    - communications, public relations, public education;
    - organizational development processes;
    - motivating and engaging clients as partners;
    - identifying and working with strengths; supporting self sufficiency and responsibility;
    - worker self management/decentralized decision making and community governance?

Individuals usually come to the point of implementing a vision because they are "called" and are compelled to do whatever is required to make it happen. For example, one director became committed to such a vision after a soul searching and an "up close look" at the daily operation of his department. His beliefs about how staff and clients should be treated were so different from the way they were being treated that he had to change the department or give up his career.

Redefining Ourselves and Our Roles

A second major decision involves determining how we personally will participate in day-to-day change efforts and how involved we will be in overseeing the efforts required to transform our departments. For example, will we be out front, highly visible and attached to this effort? Or, will we delegate this responsibility to a high level person who can handle the day to day planning, communicating, and implementing and provide the support necessary for success?

Most directors of social service departments are so busy that they have few opportunities to observe how their departments are working, how workers' needs are changing, and how clients are treated. Most directors work under incredible pressures and spend much of their time on budgetary crises, smoothing relations with the Board of Supervisors, and coping with state and federal officials. Middle managers and their supervisors handle day-to-day operations. Even middle managers are not always clear about how their clients move from intake to termination and what services look like from the clients' perspectives.

It is essential that directors find ways to understand more fully how their organization functions, what must be changed, and how it would function if it were truly a client-centered, community-based, integrated system of support for families. This does not mean that the director needs to micro-manage the operation, but time must be spent on understanding what is going on before identifying strategic opportunities for improving service delivery. In Contra Costa County it made a big difference that two of the County Supervisors and the County Administrator were 100% invested in this endeavor and knew the details of what was going on.

Planning for Implementation

After struggling with the issues of assessing one's commitment and re-defining one's role, one can turn to the hard work of planning and preparing for the implementation requirements. The actual work of implementing the vision is akin to flying a plane while making design improvements, knitting a sweater while wearing it, or renovating a house while living in it. In order to get started, Contra Costa County found it worked best to create a neighborhood-based system of service integration within and parallel to the existing county operations. In this way a "micro world" could be created for learning and testing how to do this work. This approach is less risky than throwing the entire department into upheaval; however, one must be comfortable with operating in two different and sometimes conflicting worlds at the same time. Also, one must be vigilant that this experiment is not just another project with no tie to real policy. Everything learned must be connected to improving services county-wide or else stakeholders will lose faith.

Staff must be found within the department that can work on two interdependent efforts–that of building a new infrastructure to support neighborhood services and that of community organizing and mobilizing. An individual who is very good at action planning and program and systems design, who knows the county services and how these fragmented services must be restructured, is not always the best person to work in a community involving community residents and clients in neighborhood improvement. But, the two efforts are mutually supportive and must operate with common agreement about priorities and expected results.

There are four sets of tasks that must be addressed in this planning stage. These include: (1) developing the programmatic frameworks and infrastructure for supporting community-based work; (2) determining how to obtain active community participation and partnership; (3) creating staff "buy-in" and ensuring staff success; and (4) building intra- and inter-organization collaboration. The elements of each are noted as follows:

Program Infrastructure

- Adopting prevention-oriented service models;
- Creating a unified, coherent management information system;
- Obtaining county, state and federal waivers;
- Building a management structure for operating decentralized teams;
- Developing community-focused budgets, which reflect blended funding sources.

Community Development

- "Unlearning" the past and building trust;
- Supporting the creation of neighborhood leadership;
- Clarifying community priorities;
- Creating a local governance structure;
- Bolstering self-help and mutual assistance;
- Employing neighborhood residents;
- Directing funds to community-identified priorities.

Staff Development

- Building trust and developing vision;
- Facilitating consensus on vision and values;
- Ensuring appropriate skills and competencies.

Collaboration

- Creating partnerships between county departments;
- Forging links with local businesses, funders, civic organizations and community-based organizations.

The successful accomplishment of these tasks requires certain organizational and leadership qualities. The organization must be a "learning organization" that uses data and information to correct operations. It must be organized to learn by doing, utilizing information from the management information system to improve day-to-day practice. In addition, the organization must replace protecting the department's image with a willingness to take risks and learn from mistakes, and it must ensure that everyone involved feels responsible for success and shares a comparable personal vision. Organizational leadership qualities that are required include "walking the talk," an ability to make and communicate decisions that are consistent with the vision. The leader must function as a cheerleader and rewarder, creating and providing incentives, as an educator, motivator, sales person and mobilizer. He or she must practice persistence, perseverance, and patience, be willing to "make it up as you go," and correct mistakes with little rancor. Most importantly, the leader must clearly and constantly communicate successes, lessons, and implications of changes as they occur.

Moving from Planning to Action

The action steps which must be undertaken to transform an existing system into a family-centered neighborhood human service system can be overwhelming. However, success can occur if all those involved work together with a well-organized action plan. Multiple activities and tasks can be carried out simultaneously and within common time frames if all agree on the operational plan for dividing up the tasks and responsibilities. For example, in Contra Costa County, the entire process from beginning to test-pilot stage took three-and-a-half years by taking small steps, one day at a time, which produced significant progress.

Figure 1 outlines elements of the four action areas that needed to come together to ensure project success. Each of these areas involved a number of specific action steps that kept the project moving forward to create an effective systems-level change. All were interactive and moved forward with overlapping time frames.

Establishing the vision involved educating and informing as well as listening and soliciting feedback at many levels within the County and the community. Participants needed to be allowed and assisted to articulate their reservations as well as their enthusiasm in order to develop and affirm their ongoing support. Developing the program infrastructure encompassed the "nuts and bolts" of program planning, while creating the community action plan and building the collaborative teams involved the promotion of strong and effective working relationships between individuals and organizations. The community action plan process required facilitating mutually-supportive working relationships between the neighborhood governance structure, schools, agencies and residents. The collaborative team building process focused on effective working relationships between

Figure 1. Project Action Steps

Establishing a Shared Vision and Agreeing on Desired Outcomes
- Obtain commitment from the Board of Supervisors, County Administrator, other department heads and school administrators;
- Educate management and staff about the strategic plan and common vision;
- Involve all relevant advisory boards, community coalitions, schools and community-based organizations;
- Assess the current operating processes for serving clients and identify elements that are inconsistent with a neighborhood-based, family-centered approach;
- Work with the state to eliminate regulations and finance systems that impede the new strategic direction.

Developing Program Infrastructure
- Select neighborhoods based upon defensible criteria;
- Assess needs and share information sharing about the new partnership;
- Develop a process for instituting local governance;
- Identify and recruit local leaders;
- Investigate funding streams;
- Develop management information systems, budgets, and management structures;
- Develop client consent and participation forms and procedures;
- Select staff;
- Begin joint training and staff development;
- Place the county service teams into the neighborhood.

Creating a Community Action Plan
- Facilitate the development of mutually-supportive working relationships between the neighborhood governance structure, schools, agencies, and residents;
- Monitor interactions to ensure movement toward a common set of program objectives and outcomes;
- Engage partners in developing the program infrastructure;
- Assist partners in developing a common community plan that specifies outcomes to be achieved, performance expectations, a monitoring process, and each partner's roles and responsibilities for achieving success.

Building Collaborative Teams
- Monitoring relationship building;
- Providing mediation and problem solving support "on-call";
- Resolving client-specific problems;
- Involving participants in training activities in the community;
- Promoting neighborhood opportunities to celebrate progress, life-cycle events, and holidays for children.

neighborhood center staff and clients and community members. A final step involved the selection of a neutral party to evaluate the efforts and communicating with all parties to improve the quality of life in the neighborhood.

These steps are only highlights of a complex process of systems change. Much of the change process involves exploring uncharted territory. Once a vision is developed and key leaders adapt it as part of their own personal quest, the journey begins; however, it has no predictable end point. Much of the progress made and speed of the change process will depend upon the process used to bring people together, the personalities of key individuals, success in focusing participants' energies on joint, positive action, and, of course, seizing unusual opportunities as they present themselves. If leaders have a great deal of energy, are passionate about this work, have good partners, and are patient and persistent, it can be done. Staff reported that working in the neighborhood Family Resource Center is the most difficult work they have ever done, but it is also the most meaningful. Over and over again staff report such comments as, "This is the first time in 16 years I actually enjoy coming to work everyday." Workers believe they are making a difference in the lives of their clients. Clients reported that they are shocked by the difference in the way they are treated. Many for the first time are served in a helpful, respectful manner.

THE CONSULTANT'S ROLE IN FACILITATING CHANGE

There are many different definitions of what a consultant is and what a consultant does. To some, a consultant is an expert who helps people clarify their intentions, helps design a process for achieving the organization's goals, and coaches everyone through an implementation process.

Each consultant also brings a value system and, in this case, a commitment to neighborhood-based, family-centered, inter-agency service integration. This involves promoting community participation in all aspects of neighborhood life and insuring that resources are distributed consistent with the needs and wants of the neighborhood.

The consultant's role changes over time in response to the presenting needs and requirements of the job. There were three phases of the work in Contra Costa County:

- The start up phase or the visioning process;
- The implementation planning and designing of a new system;
- Beginning operation of the pilot.

During the first phase, the consultant was responsible for drafting the vision, the set of operating principles and the strategic plan. The consultant was charged with gaining commitment and "buy in" from multiple agencies, levels in the organizations, communities, and decision makers. This was a full time job of motivating, communicating and listening to many different groups. During this stage, all of the disparate interests had to be brought into some form of agreement about the future. The consultant along with the YSB was identified with the effort, but it was the consultant's responsibility to keep everyone moving forward together.

Once the Board of Supervisors passed a Board Order in December 1992 mandating community-based, family-centered, inter-agency service integration teams to be located in the two neighborhoods of North Richmond and Bay Point, the Service Integration Management Team (SIMT) was created. As a result, the neighborhoods became associated with a larger group of concerned people, representing the departments and programs.

The consultant was the technical expert to the SIMT and helped guide the implementation planning process, structuring the work committees, overseeing the participation of all departments in making decisions, communicating with various county departments and coordinating with parallel projects related to neighborhood services. It was the consultant's responsibility to be well-informed about all of the possible methods for structuring service integration and to know and understand the "state of the art" information about the myriad of infrastructure issues that had to be dealt with (for example, financing, management information systems, self-managed teams, and evaluation) and tracked through written records of the plan, time lines, accomplishments and agreements. The consultant was a cheerleader that kept the process moving forward, serving as an activist in the community-building process and responsible for much of the day to day work of assisting the Healthy Start planning efforts, developing the North Richmond MAC, and creating communication channels between the community and the SIMT.

With the launch of the neighborhood family service centers, the County appointed a high level manager responsible for the operation and management of the neighborhood pilots. The consultant became more of an observer to the operation and shifted to a liaison role between the county and outside parties (foundations and state agency representatives), making the necessary connections to resources and expertise that could facilitate the full operation of the neighborhood centers. Specifically, the consultant conducted a technical review of all programs to determine which state and federal waivers were required to support service integration. This was done in collaboration with the County Administrator's analyst who was completing a full scale review of the existing financing mechanism and making recommendations for actions needed to maximize existing funding sources and waivers required to blend categorical funds to support the service integration efforts.

During all three steps the consultant was the person who reminded everyone about the shared vision, since everyone had many other priorities throughout the change process. The consultant maintained the county's memory on this entire enterprise and ensured communication links to the many different people who needed to be included.

The greatest challenge was coping with the slow pace of the change process. This was the consultant's only assignment, and she wanted everything to happen now. Her preferred pace was impossible for department management staff who had many competing demands on their time and energy. Allowing others a more relaxed pace, while maintaining the forward motion of the project was an ongoing balancing act.

In reviewing this experience, it seems that the consultant may have two major advantages over the appointment of an internal department manager when helping the county plan and implement neighborhood service integration. A consultant has the freedom and opportunity to speak his or her "own opinion about the truth of the circumstances" to upper management, the Board of Supervisors and the children's advocates without fear of reprisal. The consultant holds a neutral position with respect to any department or particular discipline; he/she is not required to promote the interest or defend the reputation of one department over another.

In a bureaucracy, middle managers, supervisors, and front line workers often find it difficult to say exactly what they think to upper management. Usually there are limited opportunities for their opinions to be heard and included in upper management discussions and when there is a chance to speak one's views, many worry about the repercussions of speaking up or being overly candid. Staff from different departments often reflect different organizational cultures and "ways of doing things." Even when they find it difficult to rationalize the decisions of their superiors, they are often expected or personally believe that they should present their department's "best possible face."

In contrast, the consultant's job is to present as truthfully as possible an impartial view of the circumstances and a thorough analysis of the options for action. At times, during this particular project, the consultant's opinions about what should be done in negotiations with the unions, departments and community were ignored. She walked a fine line between pushing a position that was vital to the success of the effort and accepting that others may actually better understand what is best for the program.

She learned from her mistakes as to which decisions required more persuasion and which circumstances needed an accepting, open attitude. This is a luxury which a consultant can indulge more easily than a civil servant.

The consultant is often alone when presenting an unpopular view. When staff see that upper management's response to unpleasant facts is constructive, then agency staff become more actively involved by seeing how safe it is to advocate for change.

A second advantage of hiring a consultant is that the county can hire one person who has the skills and experience required to work with both public agencies and neighborhood advisory groups. While most departments have staff who could perform in either arena, they are more than likely functioning in job classifications and current assignments which make them invisible or inaccessible to upper management. Many eligibility workers are community leaders in their neighborhoods. Many front line supervisors have learned how to get different agencies to work together when serving the same client. However, it is uncommon for a public agency to search through the bureaucracy and find these people and reassign them to a team to work inside and outside the organization. Most social services departments do not function with the kind of flexibility needed to maximize the talents and abilities of employees, regardless of classification and formal education.

CONCLUSIONS

In Contra Costa County, the process of integrating services has caused some very dramatic changes in thinking and in practice. At the beginning of the change process, no one knew how it would end up or how it would look, and no one really knew exactly how to manage the process. The project was successful because participants learned to share a strong, sustained commitment to the vision of community-based, family-centered, inter-agency service integration over an extended period of time. This commitment led to shared planning, shared operations, and mutually supportive communication. Changing the system required the following critical elements:

- Commitment and leadership from the top levels of county government were needed to keep the process on track. Commitment and leadership from the community were necessary to keep the system changes responsive to the neighborhood's needs and to mobilize local participation and ownership.
- At least one person, in this case an outside consultant, was needed to keep an eye on the larger picture, bridge gaps and keep the dialogue

open, thereby keeping everyone working together toward a shared goal.

- New ways of thinking about government, communities, workers, purposes, and service provision were needed, along with a thorough understanding of the technical information available on systems change and systems improvements.
- Participants in the process recognized the need to celebrate small changes as precursors to a larger change.

Assessing a Family-Centered Neighborhood Service Agency: The Del Paso Heights Model

Catherine Minicucci, EdM

SUMMARY. The author describes the Del Paso Model, a neighborhood-based integrated services effort underway in Sacramento County, California. Del Paso Heights is a community made up of African American, Asian, and white families on the northern side of the City of Sacramento. The County of Sacramento selected Del Paso Heights as a location to pilot a new family-centered holistic way to serve families under county human services programs in a Neighborhood Services Agency. The Del Paso Heights model demonstrates the power of the neighborhood as a focal point of integration of services and how the neighborhood can be used as a concept to overcome bureaucratic turf. Like many other community initiatives, measuring the outcomes of the Del Paso Heights Model re-

---

Catherine Minicucci is an Evaluation Consultant with Minicucci Associates, 1608 I Street, Suite 100, Sacramento, CA 95814.

The author acknowledges the role of Arthur Bolton, Director of The Center for Integrated Services, in designing the evaluation strategy.

The evaluation research was supported by grants from The Stuart Foundation, The Zellerback Family Fund, and The County of Sacramento, and was conducted in collaboration with The Center for Integrated Services for Families and Neighborhood (an institute in the Western Consortium for Public Health, affiliated with the University of California at Berkeley).

[Haworth co-indexing entry note]: "Assessing a Family-Centered Neighborhood Service Agency: The Del Paso Heights Model." Minicucci, Catherine. Co-published simultaneously in *Administration in Social Work* (The Haworth Press, Inc.) Vol. 21, No. 3/4, 1997, pp. 127-143; and: *Human Services Integration* (ed: Michael J. Austin) The Haworth Press, Inc., 1997, pp. 127-143. Single or multiple copies of this article are available for a fee from The Haworth Document Delivery Service [1-800-342-9678, 9:00 a.m. - 5:00 p.m. (EST). E-mail address: getinfo@haworth.com].

mains an elusive goal. *[Article copies available for a fee from The Haworth Document Delivery Service: 1-800-342-9678. E-mail address: getinfo@haworth.com]*

This report from the field describes progress being made in a Sacramento County, California, neighborhood known as Del Paso Heights relating to the delivery of family-centered human services. It is organized from the perspective of an outside evaluation (Brown, 1995; Colton, 1995) into three parts: (1) a description of the Del Paso Heights neighborhood and service model; (2) highlights from an assessment of the model after two years of operation; and (3) identification of some of the lessons learned about integrating human services at a neighborhood level.

DEL PASO HEIGHTS NEIGHBORHOOD SERVICE AGENCY

Del Paso Heights is a well-defined community located in the northern part of the city and county of Sacramento. In 1990, there were 10,862 residents, of whom 48 percent were African American, 23 percent white, 11 percent Hispanic, 16 percent Asian and Pacific Islanders (primarily Hmong from Laos), and 2 percent American Indian. The African American community includes a core of older homeowners who have lived in the community for a long time. The community first developed as a low income, racially mixed area of workers for the World War II Sacramento defense industry.

Del Paso Heights is home to a large number of low-income people. It has three times the rate of welfare dependency, poverty, and unemployment as the county of Sacramento as a whole. Crime rates are three to four times higher than state and national crime rates (Kelley, 1994). Teen pregnancy, low birthweight babies, and babies born exposed to illegal drugs occur at a much higher rate than in the county or state as a whole. Del Paso Heights has the highest concentration of children involved with Children's Protective Services and/or living in foster care in the county of Sacramento. Public expenditures for welfare, schools, police, fire protection and health care average $3,480 per person living in the neighborhood (Minicucci Associates, 1995a). In spite of these social and economic problems, residents talk about the closeness of the neighborhood and the fact that people know and look out for one another (Sacramento County, 1994). There are churches, schools, and recreation centers around which community life centers. The neighborhood has very few boarded up houses or graffiti covered walls due, in part, to the diligence of the Sacramento

Housing and Redevelopment Agency and the neighborhood Redevelopment Advisory Committee that oversees its work in Del Paso Heights.

In 1992, the county identified Del Paso Heights as a promising site for a neighborhood-based integrated services in the form of The Neighborhood Services Agency (NSA), featuring comprehensive, family-centered human services to increase residents' economic self-sufficiency and reduce their dependence on public assistance. With the leadership of the former chair of the Sacramento County Board of Supervisors, Grantland Johnson, opportunities emerged to restructure human services and create neighborhood service systems in connection with Sacramento County's reorganization of different human service departments and the interest of the university-connected Center for Integrated Services for Families and Neighborhoods (CISFAN).

The outcome of the county reorganization process included three elements: (1) adoption of nine principles for change, (2) reorganization of county human services into three departments, and (3) launching three new pilot projects to test a new approach to delivery of human services. The following nine principles captured the county's human services philosophy: (1) Enable people to have the highest quality of life possible; (2) Preserve and strengthen the family and/or support systems of choice; (3) Make access to services easy so that people can get the help they need; (4) Provide multidisciplinary services to multiproblem clients to focus on preservation and support of the family at the neighborhood level; (5) Assist clients in achieving and maintaining economic self-support and self-sufficiency to the extent possible, to reduce dependency on the system; (6) Move to a more generic, holistic approach to services by eliminating divisions of services that artificially categorize problem; (7) Emphasize personal responsibility; (8) Recognize that prevention is preferable to reaction; and (9) Require that programs be held accountable through research and evaluation (O'Farrell, 1994).

The Sacramento County Departments of Health and Social Services were reorganized into three new departments: Human Assistance, Health and Human Services, and Medical Systems. The new Department of Human Assistance (DHA) had responsibility for AFDC (Aid to Families with Dependent Children), General Assistance, Food Stamps, Medi-Cal eligibility, GAIN (Greater Avenues for Independence) (job training), and the community services (senior services and homeless assistance) previously administered by the Sacramento Housing and Redevelopment Agency (SHRA). The new Department of Health and Human Services had responsibility for Child Welfare Services, Public Health, and Child Health and Disability Prevention Services. The Department of Medical Systems had responsibility for medical care for the indigent, emergency services, and jail health services.

With the assistance of Arthur Bolton, who directed the Center for Integrated Services for Families and Neighborhoods (CISFAN), a neighborhood-based model was developed to include: neighborhood governance, comprehensive services, self-help and mutual assistance, and the evaluation of change in community health and well-being. The goal was to use multidisciplinary teams to assist all neighborhood families, not just existing service recipients, in achieving their economic and personal goals.

Planning for the Neighborhood Services Agency (NSA) began in July 1992 and involved agency managers, a non-profit agency director, and staff of the County Executive's Office. After hiring and training staff, the Neighborhood Services Agency was opened in March, 1993 on a busy thoroughfare at the northern end of Del Paso Heights in a county facility which also houses an AFDC bureau, Child Welfare Services Family Maintenance Bureau and Children's Protective Services units, and a primary health care clinic. The NSA has a separate door from the other two county offices in the building and is marked with a large sign designating the Neighborhood Services Agency. It includes private offices, conference space, and a welcoming reception area with couches and chairs, and toys for children, and posted on the walls are a number of job announcements, training opportunities, and bulletins about a wide range of community services. A glass partition separates the clerical reception staff from the public. In order to be admitted to the office area, a staff person must punch in a security code into a keypad near the door. The close physical proximity to existing county offices raised issues among the community residents about the lack of NSA's independent identity for delivering neighborhood-based services. In addition, it became difficult to limit services to the Del Paso Heights neighborhood when residents from outside the neighborhood requested assistance. The target area for the Del Paso Heights Neighborhood Service Agency lies within Zip Code 95838 which covers two neighborhoods, Del Paso Heights and Rio Linda, and agencies assigning staff to NSA were not consistent in using Zip Codes to limit the assignment of clients to just those in the Del Paso Heights neighborhood.

The NSA staff provided services related to drug and alcohol dependence, child health, and disability prevention, income maintenance, child protective services, and job training. Neighborhood residents who received more than one NSA service were assigned to a newly developed Multidisciplinary Team (MDT). As of June, 1995, an estimated total of 550 AFDC and GA (General Assistance) cases were served by the NSA

(16% of the cases in the target area), and the MDT had a caseload of 85 individuals and families.

In June 1995, there were 22 staff members located at the NSA. There were two managers: the Site Coordinator, with overall responsibility for NSA, and the Eligibility Supervisor, who supervises the welfare Eligibility Workers, along with two clerks. NSA staff who do not report to the Eligibility Supervisor (the social workers, GAIN staff, nurse, probation officer, etc.) also report to their parent agency supervisor in addition to the Del Paso Heights NSA Site Coordinator. The Site Coordinator reports to a Bureau Chief in the Department of Human Assistance. Eighty percent of the NSA staff volunteered for the assignment and expressed a high level of commitment to modifying the delivery of human services to assist in improving the Del Paso Heights community.

As of June 1995, the MDT process is guided by the Site Coordinator, who reviews case records regularly and meets with all NSA staff three times a week to confer on cases. In a typical meeting, the lead worker (such as the Eligibility Work or Family Maintenance social worker) describes progress to date and a second team member from a different discipline (such as the public health nurse) reports on family health related issues. Other staff might inquire about the need for additional services and a referral. The lead worker is responsible for follow-up as well as prospects for case termination and/or continuing difficulties. The MDT is focused on the neighborhood resident (sharing progress, generating ideas, and identifying needs) and is also staff-focused (peer support and problem-solving related to professional disagreements about how to work with a family).

The Mutual Assistance Network of Del Paso Heights

To address the self-help and mutual assistance goals of the NSA, a neighborhood association of residents, called the Mutual Assistance Network (MAN), was launched with the help of the staff (project director and two graduate social work interns) of the Center for Integrated Services for Families and Neighborhoods (CISFAN). The MAN Board of Directors include neighborhood residents, NSA staff, and DHA managers. As of June 1995, the MAN had nine employees and five programs, and is a provider of family support services for juvenile delinquency prevention. MAN programs include: two community gardens; a parents' support group; Asian parents' support group; grandparents' support group; a support group for children raised by grandparents; an economic development project; and a volunteer exchange.

By January 1995, the Department of Human Assistance had entered into a formal agreement with the Board of Directors of the Mutual Assistance Network of Del Paso Heights to be the advisory committee for the NSA as of July 1, 1995. The MAN Board of Directors meets formally as an Advisory Committee to the NSA with representatives of the NSA at least four times each year. The NSA may request advice from the Advisory Committee on program evaluation; evaluation, selection, and deployment of personnel; budget; future program plans; agency policies; grievances of customers; relationships with other agencies; and public relations. The agreement states that both organizations, the NSA and the MAN, are independent of one another and that MAN board members and neighborhood residents are free to advocate change in NSA policies or practices, and that the NSA is not obliged to take the Advisory Committee's advice. The agreement will be reviewed annually.

MAN's most recent efforts (1996) focus on economic development, which would involve neighborhood residents in building a neighborhood facility (with assistance from SHRA) which would house the Del Paso Heights NSA, the Del Paso Heights Elementary School District offices (currently located outside the neighborhood), and MAN itself. Additional space will be available for commercial ventures with rental income to support MAN programs.

ASSESSMENT AFTER TWO YEARS OF OPERATION

From its inception, the Del Paso Heights model of integrated services emphasized community control over decision making regarding public services. In the early discussions about neighborhood-based services, an ambitious form of community governance was envisioned. It included a governing body that would take responsibility for creating a community plan, designing and administering NSA services, hiring an Executive Director for the NSA, advocating on behalf of the residents, conducting hearings to resolve neighborhood grievances, and evaluating the quality of the NSA services.

The NSA board would be made up of elected officials, (county supervisor, city council member, state assembly member, school board members from the elementary and high school districts in the area), a representative of the County Human Services Cabinet, the chair of the Redevelopment Advisory Committee, and seven appointed neighborhood representatives.

The far reaching vision of community governance set forth in the original Del Paso Heights model was probably overly ambitious in retrospect and has yet to be implemented fully. It required far-reaching changes in decision making and financial controls and became too difficult to achieve in the short run. Most importantly, the community itself has not sought a comprehensive neighborhood governance structure. In fact, the idea of neighborhood governance came from outside. Community leaders are skeptical about the transfer of authority from government (local, state, and federal) to the neighborhood and seek to work outside of local government to improve the neighborhood. Those who originally conceived of the NSA governance model underestimated the extent of community alienation from government. Today, many community leaders are less suspicious of the NSA idea than at the outset but continue to engage in their own efforts outside of the purview of the government.

Linkage of the NSA with the Mutual Assistance Network has proven to be a productive partnership, especially in referrals between the NSA and MAN programs. Involvement of NSA staff in MAN activities is high, especially the MAN programs of grandparents rearing grandchildren. MAN serves as a community link to the NSA and provides a voice for community residents on priorities related to NSA. The MAN provides a flexible, non-governmental mechanism for neighbors to identify problems and create their own solutions.

Effective Leadership

The NSA has encountered implementation issues with leadership at all levels. Despite the support from the top leaders of the county when the pilots were launched, inevitable disagreements and problems have arisen.

The role of the County Executive's Planning Evaluation Development (PED) staff was critical in the formative stages of the Del Paso Heights NSA. They played a leadership role in the conceptualization, planning, early implementation, and evaluation strategy for the NSA. PED staff also played a very constructive role in assisting staff with the development of the MDT. The Department Managers and County Executive staff, however, did not focus sufficiently on the need to delineate clear roles and responsibilities in NSA management as they proceeded from planning to implementation. For example, many managerial leadership issues arose during the first two years of implementation. Two individuals have held the demanding position of NSA Site Coordinator, which calls for supervising 15-16 staff including eligibility workers and staff from other agencies. Most staff sent from other agencies had dual reporting responsibilities where one supervisor was in the NSA and the other in the headquarters agency. This arrangement created a "matrix management" structure which was new for the Department of Human Assistance. The NSA Site Coordinator was expected to engage in community outreach and forge partnerships with schools, city agencies, and other organizations in order to realize the vision of the neighborhood-based integrated services model. In the original staffing of the NSA, the Site Coordinator was an Eligibility Supervisor from the Department of Human Assistance and left after seven months. The position of Site Coordinator at the NSA was vacant for six months in the fall of 1993 and winter of 1994. The DHA Bureau Chief, with responsibility for pilot project implementation, took over the responsibility of site coordination during that period, provided stable leadership to the NSA, laid the groundwork for the new leadership team, and initiated training opportunities for NSA staff related to multidisciplinary team practice.

In April 1994, the second Site Coordinator, who had advanced professional training as a social worker, was appointed. The Site Coordinator had responsibility for the management of all except the Eligibility Workers who, in turn, were the responsibility of the Eligibility Supervisor and reported to the Bureau Chief in DHA.

The NSA implementation experience demonstrates that the demanding role of the Site Coordinator is critical to the success of neighborhood-based integrated services. The Site Coordinator must understand and share the vision of the NSA, demonstrate effective problem solving skills, create a framework within which the NSA staff can operate, and convey strong convictions about the merits of a team approach. In addition to value of clinical experience in guiding the work of the Multidisciplinary Team, the Site Coordinator needs skills in team building, conflict resolution, group facilitation, staff supervision, and community relations.

Effective Multidisciplinary Teams

The work of multidisciplinary teams is at the heart of the vision of the NSA in Del Paso Heights (Philliber Research, 1994). During the early planning phase, the prospect of many disciplines sitting down together to work with a family was viewed as a major component of service integration.

One year into implementation, staff still varied in their understanding and expectations of MDT practice. Some staff regarded it as informal brainstorming about a case, while others regarded it as the systematic definition of clearly defined roles and responsibilities. Some staff reported feeling intimidated by more highly educated NSA staff and fearful of bringing up cases because of the anticipated criticism of their ideas and performance. As a result, staff worked informally to strengthen the MDT process.

The different orientations, vocabularies, and working styles of professional staff also posed substantial barriers to effective teamwork. Professionals familiar with their own fields and colleagues who shared their philosophy and service approach were being asked to make a major change in their practice in order to work in concert with professionals from other disciplines, using the family-centered approach. For example, the in-home service orientation of social workers and nurses was different from the assertive group work service orientation of drug and alcohol counselors. While home visits and aggressive outreach to families is accepted as good practice in child welfare and public health, it was regarded as "coddling" or "enabling" the client in the culture of substance abuse treatment. Given that drug and alcohol abuse are both a symptom and a cause of problems for many Del Paso Heights residents, all MDT staff were given the opportunity for training in the area of substance abuse.

Another challenge to the MDT process was the need to clarify the role of the NSA Eligibility Worker. In the first 18 months of the NSA implementation, some of the Eligibility Workers felt overwhelmed by the large caseloads, since all the other staff had full caseloads from their own headquarters. At the same time, DHA Managers were concerned about the accuracy and timeliness of the AFDC, Food Stamps, and General Assistance eligibility work done by NSA Eligibility Workers. A major purpose for positioning Eligibility Workers in the NSA was to have them work directly with families to help empower them toward employment and self-sufficiency. This purpose had to be harmonized with the pressure to do "general social work" in MDT cases and the need to process standard AFDC paperwork and payments. One solution was to build family assessment into the federally required annual in-home interview for AFDC eligibility.

Given the heavy caseloads, many staff found little time to devote to MDT cases. As one staff member stated, "I have had to do my old job and my new job, keeping the old regimen going and creating time to do new things. It is very draining. I want more time to do intervention and advocacy and work on cases with other staff." Another staff person said, "Conflict between my old job and my new job is a continuous problem. My old assignment takes priority and I have to skip MDT meetings, which means that I can't commit to working with the schools. I often feel overwhelmed." In some cases, the Family Maintenance (FM) social worker and the Probation Officer have been able to deal with this overload situation with the help of their Department Managers who negotiated reduced caseloads for those NSA staff which freed them up for the "new style of work." Such changes took a considerable amount of time to accomplish.

Another barrier to effective MDT case management was the amount of paperwork required. Staff who perform assessments for their own programs in GAIN, drug and alcohol services, and child welfare services have a significant paperwork burden for their parent agencies. The MDT paperwork represents an "add on" to that burden, requiring handwritten forms to be filled out and duplicate caseloads. Without a single NSA intake form, reductions in paperwork and duplicate assessments could not be achieved.

In addition to paperwork, the NSA, in its first two years of operation, had not developed an information system to support family-centered work related to shared intake, assessments, or service outcomes. Integrated intake procedures were discussed and abandoned when it became clear how difficult it would be to satisfy separate agency regulations and reporting requirements. The County Executive's Planning staff devised a one-page service encounter form, but staff resistance and insufficient supervisory oversight resulted in inadequate information collected.

LESSONS LEARNED

The Del Paso Heights Neighborhood Services Agency is a "work in progress." It is by no means completed, as improvements continue to be made. This concluding section identifies some of the lessons learned so far in implementing a complex service integration system. There are clear advantages to family-centered multidisciplinary services for families in need. The neighborhood-based integrated services vision, however, is not easy or quick to achieve. Sacramento County's experience with the NSA shows that with leadership from top elected and appointed officials, and a vision of how new approaches to human services can be achieved, it takes time, patience, and resources to accomplish neighborhood-based services. It took about three years for the Sacramento Del Paso Heights NSA to move from the development of the original concept to implementing aspects of the vision.

Lesson #1: Creation of neighborhood-based integrated services required overcoming powerful institutional and professional barriers to be overcome.

Powerful institutional pressures pose barriers to neighborhood based services. Institutional barriers include the need for public agencies to be accountable to the laws that govern them, funding priorities, scarce resources, and the community. Two programs provide illustrations of this institutional pressure: GAIN and Children's Protective Services (CPS).

Greater Avenues for Independence (GAIN) is a program designed to prepare welfare recipients to work. GAIN is designed to serve long-term

AFDC recipients, parents under 24 without a high school diploma, and those whose children are about to turn 18 and who will be losing their welfare eligibility. Regulatory oversight of GAIN comes from the state and federal level, and there is no neighborhood focus. This is true at the county level as well, and Sacramento county does not receive sufficient resources to serve all GAIN eligible AFDC recipients.

GAIN county managers initially feared that workers located at the NSA would lose the esprit de corps of the GAIN program and their GAIN identity, miss the mutual support of fellow GAIN workers, fall behind in their understanding of GAIN program regulations, lose out on job development opportunities for GAIN clients available at the GAIN headquarters, and be pressured to serve clients (such as adolescents) who are not eligible for GAIN services. For these reasons, GAIN workers were placed in settings where other employment services were available for individuals who did not meet GAIN criteria. Exceptions were made at the Del Paso Heights NSA, where non-GAIN employment services were provided by two half-time (1 full-time) GAIN workers as well as a foundation-supported NSA job developer from a community-based organization who subsequently was funded by the Sacramento Employment Training Agency (SETA) under contract with the YWCA. The NSA implementation experience has demonstrated that GAIN services can be integrated in an effective manner with non-GAIN employment services in a neighborhood where job developers and GAIN workers target a specific neighborhood population.

The second example of barriers to merging existing county services with neighborhood services can be found in the area of child welfare services. There is heavy legal and public pressure on Child Welfare Services to act quickly to prevent child injury and death from abuse or neglect. Faced with 3,000 reports a month to CPS for suspected child abuse and neglect, Sacramento County can only afford to investigate 500 reports. The county investigates the most severe reports of sexual abuse, physical abuse, and severe neglect. The type of neglect commonly seen by school staff (children falling asleep in class, children who are hungry or without shoes, or children with head lice) are usually not considered complaints severe enough for CPS investigation given the level of CPS resources. These are the types of problems for which school staff want assistance from the Del Paso Heights NSA. Visits to such homes often reveal much deeper problems (commonly substance abuse and mental illness) and the neglect of children is only a symptom.

County Managers of CPS are reluctant to divert scarce resources to neighborhood-based efforts for several reasons. The first is a requirement to be able to respond quickly to emergencies wherever they occur in the county to prevent child injury or death. Children at imminent risk must be served. The second is the fear (based on previous experience) that out-stationed social workers in neighborhoods tend to be drawn into working on less severe neglect cases, putting their emphasis on prevention rather than more severe cases requiring crisis intervention. To date, resources diverted to neighborhood services have not lowered the demand in those neighborhoods for CPS services. CPS resources are stretched so thinly that they barely can handle crisis intervention. At the same time, CPS social workers are in great demand because of their skill in working with families and obtaining needed services for families. The NSA needs skilled social workers not already committed to protecting children in crisis, in order to provide the other needed services in a non-crisis environment.

In addition to the institutional pressures related to GAIN and CPS, overcoming professional barriers was another challenge. The creativity of different workers needed to be released so that staff could contribute their own talents to working with families. The eligibility workers encouraged welfare recipients to get job training and helped them find child care and transportation. The drug counselors confronted the denial of a drug user who is harming her children. The social worker simultaneously counseled with families, consulted with school staff, and coordinated other team members in helping families in crisis. The public health nurse helped families and children gain access to health care providers. The probation officer worked with parents to become better role models for their teens on probation by referring them to a member of the NSA employment services team. The GAIN worker encouraged job applicants to get a drug test and encouraged local employers to hire neighborhood residents.

Achieving a cohesive NSA team has taken time and patience on the part of Site Coordinators and DHA Managers. Commitment on the part of managers and staff members to keep trying new approaches when the team encountered obstacles was an important ingredient in successfully implementing the NSA model. Leadership was required to build a climate of trust so that staff could, admit failure, and search together for new strategies and solutions.

Lesson #2: Start-up resources for neighborhood-based integrated services need to include fun-for staff training, time for joint planning, support for information systems development, and structuring the evaluation processes.

Accomplishing fundamental change in the way public employees work with citizens requires training, new information resources, time to try new things, and new approaches to evaluation. Investment in start-up costs is critical for success. A great deal of training is needed for staff and managers to work as a team in conducting effective home visits and demonstrating effective interviewing and negotiating skills. Managers need training in conflict resolution. All staff need training in the underlying problems, such as substance abuse, that cut across all programs.

Tracking the work of the integrated services team requires a new approach to information systems development, which is different from systems designed to serve single programs. Such a system needs the capacity for single intake, on-line information sharing, tracking cases for ongoing monitoring, and reporting. Also, there is a need for agreed upon outcome measures, and regular reports to the staff, to agency managers, and county leaders on the success of the neighborhood services agency. Del Paso Heights NSA was implemented without the benefit of new approaches to information systems, and the result is a limited ability to assess the impact of the NSA on its neighborhood service recipients.

Lesson #3: Neighborhood is a powerful concept that can have a profound effect upon public decision making and on the allocation of resources, start, new services, and inter-agency collaboration.

Powerful advantages flow from the neighborhood focus. By concentrating on a neighborhood, agencies that normally work in isolation are able better to work together for the common good. As staff from different agencies get to know one another, there can be a significant improvement in communications, referrals, and jointly funded projects. NSA staff learn about the array of local services and whether or not an agency has available capacity to serve additional people. If an agency is overloaded and needs more resources, staff in other agencies can help to identify resources. For example, while the need for child care exceeded supply and there were waiting lists for Head Start, an underused private child care agency was located.

The Mutual Assistance Network and the NSA worked together to identify needs and available resources. For example, MAN identified the lack of transportation as a barrier to service. Through the Block Grandparent Program, it was found that most residents did not have access to transportation to take their children to the doctor, dentist, child care center, or enrichment activities. Since transportation became a high priority for agencies establishing new programs in Del Paso Heights, the Mutual Assistance Network purchased two vans to transport residents to programs and events.

Another advantage to a neighborhood focus is in employment of neighborhood residents by social services agencies. Agencies that want to hire community residents cooperate by sharing the pool of job applicants. Also, public employees in social services agencies who lived in Del Paso Heights were given priority in transferring to the Neighborhood Services Agency. Such employees contributed an idealism, knowledge of the community, rapport with the residents, and a sense of hope for the future, providing an intangible benefit to the NSA. These developments are part of the dynamism of the Del Paso Heights neighborhood today which did not exist five years ago, and are more powerful than agency managers miles away could easily appreciate. These changes help to make existing resources stretch further, foster creativity, and enhance the effectiveness of publicly funded programs.

Lesson 4: *When serving a prescribed geographic target area, marketing and outreach efforts are needed to inform the community about integrated services which tend to be beyond the experience and expertise of most government human service agencies.*

The evaluation of the Del Paso Heights model revealed that many of the human services staff were defining the target population more broadly than the original framers of the model intended. There appeared to be a tension between adhering to the target population within a given Zip Code and the desire to serve residents on a first come first serve basis. It was very tempting for workers and their host agency supervisors to assume responsibility for "out of area cases" rather than engaging in more marketing and outreach to the target area. It was very hard to keep the focus on the Del Paso Heights neighborhood, and apparently there was very little discussion and analysis of the problems related to reaching out to the target population.

It was understandable that the NSA would receive referrals and wanted to nurture referral relationships. NSA staff found it hard to say "no" to people in need. It was harder to seek out the people who need help but do not search for it than to accept the "seekers" who do not live in the area. The county agency staff did not share the " neighborhood" service philosophy in many cases and did not see a problem in adding a few more areas to the target population. The need for ongoing, creative marketing that is personal and tailored to the neighborhood was underestimated by the NSA managers, leaders in the county, and staff. For example, when outreach was conducted in non-traditional way by Block Grandparents going to food stamp lines or day care centers, the word about the NSA and MAN got out into the community.

Lesson #5: The location and appearance of an integrated services facility send a very important message to the community with unintended consequences.

NSA's physical location was a problem for some neighborhood residents and posed a barrier to seeking services. Many residents could not tell the difference between the regular AFDC bureau and health clinic housed in the same building as the NSA office. Location and symbolism are both important factors in marketing the integrated services concept to the neighborhood.

Lesson #6: Neighborhood-based information is essential for setting priorities, measuring progress, and mobilizing support for action.

From the earliest planning efforts, it was recognized that for outcome evaluation (supported in part by local foundations), a comprehensive neighborhood description and baseline data must be developed as a point of comparison for assessing neighborhood improvement over time. In addition, a comprehensive descriptive report on Del Paso Heights was completed in March 1995 (Minicucci Associates, 1995a). The data in both reports have been used to mobilize others. For example, there is a movement to organize on behalf of youth education and employment by neighborhood activists (using the data on the 50% graduation rates of those entering the 9th grade). Additional foundation support provided for a more in depth analysis of implementation than would otherwise have been possible with existing evaluation resources (Minicucci Associates, 1995b).

The development of neighborhood-specific information is critical to focusing on a geographic area, making apparent the connections between social problems and identifying community strengths. Sharing information across agencies about outcomes that reflect on community health and well-being has spurred collaboration among agencies and organizations. The Del Paso Heights experience suggests that neighborhood-based integrated services efforts need to pay attention to the important use of information which can focus on the totality of the community and not just on existing fragmented programs.

Others have written about practical methodological problems in assessing the outcomes of family-centered services (Connell, 1995). In Del Paso Heights, there were many commonly identified problems, including unclear goals, inadequate information systems to track the nature, extent, and duration of services, inadequately defined service outcomes, and the absence of comparison groups. Simply defining the services to be provided proved to be a monumental challenge.

Lack of information on the nature, duration, and intensity of NSA services, as well as service outcomes, remains a serious gap on the DPH model. There were no resources regularly to evaluate service outcomes, assess community outcomes, or assess outcomes for neighborhood residents who receive public services but are not part of the NSA. An overall evaluation strategy is needed that will take into account these important changes.

Lesson #7: Neighborhood-based integrated service systems need time, patience and leadership to build referral systems and collaborative services among community agencies.

The short history of the NSA illustrates that many unanticipated issues arise when promoting change in human service systems. For example, the elementary schools have worked in partnership with the NSA, referring families and jointly working on cases with school counselors and NSA staff. In general, the schools refer their most severe school attendance and underachievement cases to the NSA. The NSA has developed a system of school liaisons in which a staff member of the NSA serves as the sole point of referral for a particular school. Since the most common types of problems referred from schools to the NSA are potential neglect cases (in which a child has missed a great deal of school due to a health problem), families overwhelmed with a range of other problems, and unmet physical and health needs of children, the social worker and the public health nurse offer the most commonly needed professional services.

Schools, along with other county agencies, are complex organizations, and it has taken time for each entity to learn how to work with the NSA. As agency representatives work together on particular cases, the partnership has deepened and become mutually beneficial.

CONCLUSION

The NSA in 1996, after three years of operation, was poised to enter the second stage of its development. Extensive planning and initial implementation had been achieved. The next stage of development included: (1) locating a community facility for the NSA with its own identity; (2) expansion of the NSA services to all AFDC recipients in the target area; and (3) creation of an information system that is built upon a neighborhood focus and includes the capacity for service outcome assessment. Pioneering work in the arena of family-focused, integrated neighborhood services has many challenges and many rewards as is reflected in this case study of the teamwork found in the Del Paso Heights neighborhood of Sacramento, California.

REFERENCES

Brown, P. The role of the evaluator in comprehensive community initiatives. (1995). In J.P. Connell et al. (1995). (Eds.), *New approaches to evaluating community initiatives*. Washington, DC: Aspen Institute.

Center for Integrated Services for Families and Neighborhoods. (1992, June 24). Del Paso Heights Model. Oakland, CA: President's National Commission on America's Urban Families.

Community Services Planning Council. (1994, January). *Sacramento County Zip Code data book: Vital statistics and use of public programs*. Sacramento, CA: Community Services Planning Council.

Connell, J.P. et al. (Eds). (1995). *New approaches to evaluating community initiatives*. Washington, DC: The Aspen Institute.

Coulton, C.J. Using community level indicators of children's well-being in comprehensive community initiatives. (1995). In J.P. Connell et al. (Eds.), *New approaches to evaluating community initiatives*. Washington, DC: The Aspen Institute.

Kelly, K. (1994). *Out of control*. Boston: Addison-Wesley.

Minicucci Associates. (1995a). Del Paso Heights: Information for neighborhood based planning and evaluation. Sacramento, CA: Center for Integrated Services for Families and Neighborhoods.

Minicucci Associates. (1995b). Creating a neighborhood based system: The Del Paso Heights experience. Sacramento, CA: Center for Integrated Services for Families and Neighborhoods.

O'Farrell, J. (1994, July). Department heads' responsibility and functions of PED. Sacramento, CA: Office of the County Executive.

Philliber Research Associates. (1994, May). An evaluation of the caring communities program at Walbridge Elementary School. Accord, NY: Philliber Research Associates.

Sacramento County Department of Health and Human Services. (1994, December). The Del Paso Heights block grandparents project: Raising young children in Del Paso Heights. Sacramento, CA: DHHS.

Applications of Boundary Theory to the Concept of Service Integration in the Human Services

Alexis A. Halley, DPA

SUMMARY. Service integration (SI) is an aspect of theorizing about organizations and governance. To discover questions for future practice and theory-building, the analysis here reframes the SI concept in the human services from the typical starting point of fragmentation-integration to the imperatives of boundary theory. Extant SI discourse is a confused array of descriptive, normative, and explanatory theory. An action-reflection interplay with conflicting and missing values is revealed. Boundary spanning and boundarylessness, defined in five metaphors, illustrate boundary theory. Selected literature on SI in the human services is translated into boundary theory (e.g., types of SI boundaries, SI boundary values and roles) and a research agenda is posed. *[Article copies available for a fee from The Haworth Document Delivery Service: 1-800-342-9678. E-mail address: getinfo@haworth.com]*

The article by Hassett and Austin (1997) that opens this volume gives an important description of the history of service integration (SI) as a set

Alexis A. Halley is Senior Fellow, Executive Leadership Center, Mt. Vernon College, Washington, DC 20007; Director of the Stennis Congressional Staff Fellows Program; and Executive Director, Meridian International Institute.

The author acknowledges the useful inputs by Michael J. Austin, John J. Kirlin, and Frank P. Sherwood, in the design and implementation of this study.

[Haworth co-indexing entry note]: "Applications of Boundary Theory to the Concept of Service Integration in the Human Services." Halley, Alexis A. Co-published simultaneously in *Administration in Social Work* (The Haworth Press, Inc.) Vol. 21, No. 3/4, 1997, pp. 145-168; and: *Human Services Integration* (ed: Michael J. Austin) The Haworth Press, Inc., 1997, pp. 145-168. Single or multiple copies of this article are available for a fee from The Haworth Document Delivery Service [1-800-342-9678, 9:00 a.m. - 5:00 p.m. (EST). E-mail address: getinfo@haworth.com].

of evolving practices and emerging challenges. This paper will build on the foundation set there to examine SI from the imperatives of theory. The thesis to be developed is that SI, as a concept, needs to be reframed (e.g., Kagan & Neville, 1993; O'Looney, 1993) for the information age (e.g., Rosell, 1995) so that we have better questions to pose for future practice and theory-building.

Complaints about the status of SI as a concept have been growing in recent years. SI has been characterized as lacking in crisp language, as being, at once, a philosophy, an objective, and a set of strategies and structural arrangements, and as being difficult to separate from other strategies of service reform (e.g., Kagan & Neville, 1993; Agranoff, 1991; Yessian, 1995). The SI theoretical literature is charged with falling short, and the concept itself is regarded as too global and too prescriptive rather than analytical (e.g., Martin, Chackerian, Imershein, & Frumkin, 1983).

To begin the task of developing SI theoretically, this study advances three propositions: (1) SI is a concept deeply rooted in the practice of delivering human services; (2) SI, as a concept in the human services, lacks adequate treatment at a fundamental (explanatory) theoretical level linked to but moving beyond practice; and (3) a body of work known as boundary theory (which includes boundaries, boundary spanning, and boundarylessness) is one useful way to reframe the current SI discourse so as to link and further develop the next generation of SI theory and practice. Accordingly, the discussion has three main parts: (1) identification of the levels at which SI is currently discussed to lay a foundation for linking conceptual development of SI to boundary theory; (2) presentation of a conceptual scheme to understand key elements of boundary theory; and (3) discussion of how application of the key elements of boundary theory can potentially inform a future SI conceptual development agenda including its normative features.

SI is a textbook illustration of the caveat that concepts are basic building blocks in the process of building scientific knowledge and in the process of building actionable knowledge (Kirlin, 1984). It is only by going deeply into concepts that contemporary questions can be recast to yield a fundamentally different, and possibly more advanced type of discussion.

TWO LEVELS OF SI DISCOURSE

To begin, the extant discourse on SI can be described at two levels: (1) practice, action, or intervention (Moore, 1992), and (2) reflection or explanation (e.g., Argyris, 1970; Briar & Miller, 1971). These two levels are illustrated by the scan of ten SI articles or books noted in Table 1.

Table 1 shows that SI is grounded in human acts. The empirical (or practice) origins for SI are a wide array of reform movements, program designs, and tools directed to changing fractured human service delivery systems at policy, operating, and local (client interface) levels. The "action" side of SI contains community integration, coordinated services, comprehensive services, privatization, co-location, single intake or application procedures, case management, multi-problem clients, and cost minimization. The action side of SI also contains the descriptive history of SI in the United States, starting as early as the colonial period and the Civil War, when the use of a "service" came to be seen as a vehicle to reform deep-seated economic and social problems that transcended the neighborhood (Kagan & Neville, 1993). It is "in practice" that government creates legal categories of human need and then provides grants and launches programs targeted to specific population groups based on the legal categories (Hassett & Austin, 1997).

The human acts which constitute SI also have meaning with respect to bodies of theories and attendant values that are rarely treated as a set or on their own terms in a manner comparable to SI at the level of action. The second column of Table 1 (and elements of the first) illustrates this next "level" of the discourse on SI. The terms there suggest that the practice of SI draws from and feeds into at least the following theories, each concentrating on a different unit of analysis: federalism/governance, interorganizational and intersectoral (public-private) theories, public choice theory, institutional change and innovation, humanistic theory, and what might be characterized as an emerging "boundary theory." For example, boundary theory, has a terminology that would characterize SI as "reducing or eliminating categorical boundaries," and as seeking to promote boundary spanning designs and behaviors. This is in contrast to the discourse of federalism which portrays SI with respect to the changing role of the federal government in integrating and fragmenting human services vis-à-vis the role of state, regional, and local governments, or the discourse of interorganization theory which focuses on transorganizational systems, management and service delivery networks and configurations.

Table 1 also reveals attendant, if not implicit and even conflicting, values in this body of SI literature. Such values include, for example, an apparent rejection of benefits that might accrue from duplication and overlap (e.g., Landau, 1969); an aim for greater effectiveness of impact and outcomes of services; and a complex ideology that (1) decries fragmentation, narrow program missions, specialization, and particularization

TABLE 1. Service Integration (SI): Action and Reflection

Author	Problem in Action or Practice	Problem in Reflection or Explanation
Agranoff, 1991	Quest for policy, operating, and local systems responsive to multiple needs of persons at risk Community integration, comprehensive services, coherent services, broad spectrum of services, coordinated services	Interorganizational coordination Transorganizational systems and management
Edwards and D. Austin, 1991	The recurrent cry for more coordination among programmatically linked organizations is a reflection of the limited control and management that typically exists within service delivery networks, which have open, undefined boundaries	Service delivery networks to which human service organizations belong (external environment of human service organizations)
Hassett and M. Austin, 1997	Changing definitions of service integration over time (history of service integration) Challenges for the future	Efforts to reduce or eliminate divisions or boundaries between categorically defined and provided services Institutional change
John, Halley, and Fosler, 1996	Geographic and substantive fragmentation of human service delivery system and programs	Federalism/intergovernmental relations/ governance of fragmentation (four styles)
Kagan and Neville, 1993	History of service integration (changing definition over time, in practice)	Structuralist organization theory Open systems theory: organization-environment Federalism: Intergovernmental relations (human service obligations of a government to its citizens) Institutional change Humanistic: behavior of individuals

Author	Problem in Action or Practice	Problem in Reflection or Explanation
Kirlin, 1996	Numerous efforts to integrate services in response to complaints of fragmentation, with modest results	Debates about design How complex functional systems are bounded How government creates choice structures and values of place, complex systems, and goods and services in differentiated arenas of action
Martin, Chackerian, Imershein, and Frumkin, 1983	How to: reduce duplication, enhance coordination, minimize costs, address multi-problem client Unified administrative structure; local vs. state administrative control over line workers; case management; co-location of services across program areas; single intake or application procedure	Organizational innovation for solving duplication, fragmentation, inefficiency, unresponsiveness, etc. Ideology or grounds for social reform Three types of dimensions: structural, procedural, geographic
O'Looney, 1993	Reform movements: greater privatization vs. greater integration Both directed to changing fractured and bureaucratic system of service delivery	Market models (exit): problem, in part, is size of bureaucracy Public choice theory Voice models (not size but fracturing) Public-private relationship
Yessian, 1995	Firmly rooted service agencies, most with narrow missions focusing on particular needs Specialized human service workforce; few generalists	Linkages Institutional reform (purpose, level, mix of services, integrated delivery systems)
Weiner, 1990	Duplication and overlap in provision of services in society A nonsystem of separate, isolated agencies each providing services from own disciplinary perspective Greater effectiveness of services re: client impact and outcomes	Transorganizational management Transorganizational systems Integrated service delivery technologies Systems as networks of agencies linked together; boundary spanning Vertical and horizontal integration Levels of integration-coordination (service delivery, systems management)

of service categories in the system; yet (2) idealizes integration as particularizing a comprehensive package of services for individual consumers or clients, be they person or family; and (3) idealizes integration as coherence, comprehensiveness, and coordination in and among large systems of service delivery. It seems that SI contains a presumption that something "more unified, more integrated" (for the system and/or the consumer) is much better, and more preferred than something that is too differentiated, too fragmented, too specialized. What does it mean to say that services are too fragmented? Does a complaint about fragmentation imply that diversity is not valued? Do we want diversity of services but integration of service provision? What does it mean to argue that services need to be more integrated, especially during an emerging information society, when:

> We live in an age of increasing specialization, and for good reason. Humanity keeps learning more about each field of study; and as every specialty grows, it tends to split into subspecialties. That process happens over and over again, and it is necessary and desirable. However, there is also a growing need for specialization to be supplemented by integration. The reason is that no complex, nonlinear system can be adequately described by dividing it up into subsystems or into various aspects defined beforehand. . . . In academic life, in bureaucracies, and elsewhere, the task of integration is insufficiently respected. (Gell-Mann, 1994, p. 345)

Differentiation, diversity, and fragmentation are certainly constants in life, organizations, policies, and the like. So too are efforts to integrate. With a label like service "integration," one has the sense that something is left out, that only one side of a coin is being valued. Might it be, for example, that integration and fragmentation are both needed? Are we treating fragmentation and integration as either/or dichotomies? Might it be that the act or outcome of integration is inseparable from the act or outcome of fragmentation, differentiation, or a state of diversity? Is it not the case that under assumptions of public choice theory, for example, a rationale is provided for positive consequences of fragmentation/differentiation and less directed processes? Is SI really an argument for centralization in disguise? Add to these questions the possibility that there might be missing values to be created at human service boundaries; values such as service sustainability, for example, or service ecology, or stewardship, even as the differentiation-integration features are balanced.

An action-reflection interplay that is descriptive, normative, and explanatory is thus at the heart of the SI concept as we know it in the human services. Indeed, if knowledge-building is considered as a long-term, cyclical process, the cumulative work on SI can be construed as an extensive period of fieldwork that shows both a progression of and interplay between practice (action or intervention) and reflection (or explanation), each with embedded norms or values. The bulk of the theoretical work on SI, however, is best characterized as taking place at the level of interventive theory as opposed to explanatory theory (e.g., Briar & Miller, 1971; Argyris, 1970).

(Interventive theory is analogous to practice or action directed to coming between or among persons, groups, or objects for the purpose of helping them; it is the framework that defines what practitioners do in a particular area of work (such as SI in the human services). In the human services, intervention theory in general seeks answers to the question "how can "x" be changed (in the present case, how can "x" be integrated). Explanatory theory is developed to consider why does "x" exist or how did "x" come to be. Briar and Miller (1971) note that the questions answered for interventive theory are quite different and sometimes independent from the questions answered for explanatory theory.)

Service integration constitutes a fascinating piece of the history of theorizing about organizations and governance. Most of the SI discussion, however, is in terms of the fragmentation-integration dichotomy as the foundational question. Another category that might also be foundational is boundaries, which emerges as less developed and less familiar in extant explanatory work (e.g., from the Table 1 analysis of SI). Since boundary theory can potentially incorporate descriptive (interventive), explanatory (reflective), and normative (value) questions, boundary theory will be examined next as a background within which to explore deeper understanding of the SI concept in the human services.

KEY ELEMENTS OF BOUNDARY THEORY

Boundary is an important concept in many disciplines (Halley, 1995). It is well developed in the physical sciences and in the social and behavioral sciences, including business administration, but it is less well developed in public administration or human service administration.

Boundary is a fundamental notion, at once simple and complex, consistent and paradoxical. A boundary is a line, a region, or a zone that divides, separates, distinguishes, sets limits, or is the limit itself. Whether in the physical, behavioral, or symbolic realms, what goes on at the boundary says a great deal about what happens on either side. Boundaries are loci of highly charged contact where differences meet and exchanges occur (e.g., friction, conflict, power, ritual, and resource conversion). Boundaries may also be regarded as the perceptual arrangements we use to separate or unite, differentiate and connect ourselves to the world (Michael, 1995). They help us establish and maintain habits, rules and expectations, provide defense, allow exchange to occur, and define membership and roles. For those disciplines explicitly concerned with boundary as a formal concept (e.g., systems theory, cybernetic theory, information theory, political science, and anthropology), the focus on boundary is typically on its role as setting limits, separations, and divisions. Comparatively, less emphasis is given to what might be regarded as the interlocking nature of activity within the boundary area itself, a fact that prompted at least one social science observer to recommend that the term "interface" really ought to replace boundary, as interface expressed more the duality and exchange inherent in boundary as both a place of separation and connection (Weinberg, 1975).

Origins of Boundary Spanning and Boundarylessness

The study of boundaries examines how they emerge, develop, and disappear, how they are value-laden, and how they represent the lines of contact (concrete or symbolic) that afford opportunities for both cooperation and conflict. "Boundary theory" is a term that appears in the literature of political geography and international relations. A recent survey examining how boundary has been developed in many substantive areas (Halley, 1995) revealed that there is, indeed, a body of work that might be regarded as constituting the elements of interdisciplinary "boundary theory." Boundary theorists can be identified in economics, law, philosophy, political geography, political science, public administration, psychology, social psychology, administrative theory, and futures studies, to name a few. Their work encompasses (1) foundational work on boundaries (basic terminology, perspectives, values, methodology, and history), and (2) the dynamics of boundaries (e.g., boundary making, boundary change, conflict and power, spanning, learning, and boundarylessness).

Two conceptual perspectives, not mutually exclusive, have formed the orientation within which the term boundary takes on significance in the social and behavioral sciences and professions. The first is the systems approach or general systems theory, which considers boundaries, environments, wholes, processes, and relationships. In this context, the study of boundaries has shifted, over time, from looking at the form of boundaries and their location (i.e., structure) to the functions boundaries perform (or the functional aspects of structure), and then to the processes that are involved with boundary interaction. The second perspectives are those represented by particular areas of knowledge such as political science, and physical science. Johnston (1988) believes that the managerial approach offers the most comprehensive and least reductionist approach to boundary theory and can incorporate both general systems thinking and the knowledge of specialized disciplines.

Interest in boundaries is especially strong during times of great boundary change. For example, shortly after the two world wars, attention riveted to the redefinition of nation-state boundaries. Today, however, it is not war but the exponential increase in information, made possible in part by information technology, that is shifting, blurring, and otherwise challenging the dominant mythologies which are maintained and expressed by boundaries–whether physical, ideological, factual, procedural, organizational, programmatic, personal, or relational. Today, Michael (1995) argues that the important boundaries are "... determined less by material circumstances such as geography and more by concepts, relationships, and flows of information in the form of money and other symbols" (p. 3). Similarly, Rosell (1995) believes that the emergence of a global information society is accelerating the pace of change and overwhelming established methods of governing and organizing that were developed for a world of more limited information flow, greater stability, and clearer boundaries.

Boundary spanning is a term that has strong roots in the open systems literature of business administration and management. Boundary spanning, at heart, is a process or behavior that occurs across boundaries. At the *individual* level, boundary spanning has been defined as persons who operate as exchange or linking agents at the periphery or boundary of the organization with elements outside it (Leifer & Huber, 1977) and who link two or more systems whose goals and expectations are likely partially conflicting (Miles, 1980). At the *organizational* level, boundary spanning is defined more as organizational systems that manage social, task, and institutional environments, and that filter, protect, buffer, and represent the organization to its environment (Adams, 1983). At the *transorganization* level, boundary spanning refers to the interaction processes within and among networks of organizations (a logical type higher than that of single organizations) working to resolve macro problems which could not be solved by organizations acting alone (Cummings, 1984). Boundary spanning is anchored in classical, rational-analytic, systems thinking that makes a clear differentiation between an organization and its environment.

Boundary spanning was popular in the 1970s and 1980s, at least in the organizational literature. During the late 1980s and early 1990s, the term boundarylessness (or boundaryless) has surfaced to describe a "new" way of doing business across boundaries in and among organizations. Most accounts attribute its practical origins to Jack Welch at General Electric (G.E.) who, when he became CEO, said he wanted G.E. to become a "boundaryless" organization, where "we knock down the walls that separate us from each other on the inside and from our key constituencies on the outside" (Hirschhorn & Gilmore, 1992). In that sense, and in others as well, boundaryless is similar to SI in that the latter gained some popularity (and spawned a great deal of practice and literature) when Elliott Richardson announced it as one of his initiatives at H.E.W.:

> Service integration is ways of organizing the delivery of services to people at the local level. SI is . . . a process aimed at developing an integrated framework . . . (I)ts objectives must include such things as: (a) the coordinated delivery of services for the greatest benefit to people, (b) a holistic approach to the individual and family unit, (c) provision of a comprehensive range of services locally, and (d) rational allocation of resources at the local level to be responsive to local needs. (Quoted in Yessian, 1995)

Boundarylessness has three features: (1) an aggressive undertaking (knocking down walls), (2) a collaborative activity (create shared goals), and (3) a synthetic exercise (integrated diversity). As in boundary spanning, the idea is to bridge differences, but in doing so, not to be protecting turf but to be consciously blurring turf. The results might be higher levels of integration, a seamless government or delivery system, flexible work, and continuous innovation. Equally, the effort might produce boundary violation, codependence, and overly rigid boundaries. In organizational and leadership realms, boundaryless is regarded as a way of managing based on information such that distinctions (boundaries) do not get in the way of transferring knowledge, services, and goods in the most efficient way possible (Devanna & Tichey, 1990).

Five Metaphors to Characterize Boundary Spanning and Boundaryless

Boundary spanning and boundarylessness are cross-level constructs—units of analysis on their own terms, each of which integrates information across multiple levels of data and explanation (Halley, 1995). As such, they operate at the level where one describes meta-concepts that work across the familiar hierarchical units of individual, group, or organization (e.g., Caldwell, 1994). To illustrate this property, the literature on boundary spanning and boundarylessness can be characterized according to five metaphors: organizational adaptation, learning and innovation processes, leadership and power, psychological properties, and design of complex systems (see Table 2 for a summary of key themes). Drawing upon Table 2, boundary spanning and boundaryless themes in each metaphor can be briefly summarized as follows.

Organizational Adaptation. Applied to *boundary spanning*, theorists and researchers discuss organization-environment interactions which adapt or fail to adapt the organization to its environment. Most emphasize the boundary spanning role or position, operating distinct from the stable core of productive activity (Thompson, 1967). Boundary spanning is carried out differently depending on the organizations involved (Leifer, 1975), and boundary spanners have been shown to be more influenced by the nature of their work goals than by their manager's behavior (Robertson, 1995). *Boundarylessness* describes the organizational form (basically transparent internal and internal-external boundaries) that enables ongoing adaptation: rapid response to customer needs and to conditions of a turbulent environment (Bergquist, 1993). Information technology will be a main force bringing organizations together, thus creating transparent boundary conditions among organizations and much greater needs for interorganizational effectiveness (Davidson & Davis, 1990). As old boundaries are dropped, a crisis of familiar organizational boundaries and missions ensues (Bergquist, 1993).

Learning/Information/Innovation. Applied to *boundary spanning*, boundaries are crucial sites for learning and innovation, determined today by concepts and information flows, but communication across boundaries is extraordinarily inefficient and prone to bias and distortion (Tushman, 1977). Institutions matter because of the boundaries they create. In a foreground of rapid change, there will be a continuing mismatch between institutions and the boundaries they create (Schon, 1971). Society and government need to learn how to continually develop new procedures to span the increasingly complex sectoral, intergovernmental, interagency, interprogram, and interlevel boundaries as well as the conceptual, temporal, and symbolic boundaries (Michael, 1995). *Boundarylessness* identifies learning organizations, learning systems, social transformation and values. Boundaryless organizations compete on speed and learning rather than specialization and economies of scale (Devanna & Tichey, 1990). To do that, they must be self-renewing organizations, with more democratic processes that involve all levels of the workforce in disseminating knowledge, goods, and services. This means reframing how we think about organizations, shifting from a rational-bureaucratic mode to a learning systems mode (Schon, 1971). The informatization of society has disintegrative effects, so new ways of integrating (learning systems based ap-

TABLE 2. Five Metaphors for Boundary Spanning and Boundarylessness (Halley, 1995)

Metaphor	Applied to Boundary Spanning Literature	Applied to Boundarylessness Literature
Organizational Adaptation	• Organization adapts or fails to adapt to changes in environment through behavior of those who operate across organization-environment boundary • Boundary spanning differs from productive core • Boundary spanners more influenced by work goals than by manager's behaviors • Represent and protect organization; information gatekeeper vis-à-vis external environment • Differences in doing boundary spanning across organizations	• Organizational responsiveness to customers • Interorganizational effectiveness • Ongoing adaptation • Mission and boundary crises • Educators (teach people what boundaries matter most, manage paradox, seek out and engage environmental turbulence, facilitate feedback from environment and between organizational subgroups)
Learning/ Information/ Innovation	• Boundaries are crucial sites for learning and innovation; need continual learning to span boundaries • Boundaries determined by concepts, relationships, flows of information • Institutions matter because of the boundaries they create • Continuing mismatch between institutions and the boundaries they create • Boundary spanners who can reach across boundaries • Boundary communication inefficient and prone to bias and distortion	• Compete on speed and learning rather than on specialization and economies of scale • Holism, integration for customer outcomes • Relationship between boundaries (e.g., center-periphery) and organizational learning • Informatization of society • Boundary spanners with common language to enable communication across boundaries • Boundary spanning (learning) infrastructure • Searching, exploring attitude; shifting center

Metaphor	Applied to Boundary Spanning Literature	Applied to Boundarylessness Literature
Leadership/ Power	• Leadership located at the borders where there is a break in the system (horizontal and vertical) • Ambassador and interpreter of external environment to home base organization, with decreasing capacity to influence events within that organization • Boundary spanning role has two independent roles: gatekeeper and representative • Map situations in terms of strategy, operations, tactics	• Outmoded language of leadership due to informatization of society • Aggressive, horizontal leadership to blur, break down hierarchical boundaries • Boundary path of exchange leadership • See and address "new" invisible (psychological) boundaries • Theory crisis
Psychological Aspects	• Psychological boundaries in relationships • Boundaries contain anxiety and uncertainty • Subjective boundaries do not correspond always to formal organizational boundaries • Draw appropriate boundaries • Pre-modern/modern psyche: embedded in tradition, ethics based on principles, collaborate only when necessary, contain anxiety through reason, power, self-mastery	• Transition to global information society (rather than being there) precipitates different psychological boundary responses: • Global neurosis: rigidify boundaries (them-us, win-lose) • Global psychosis: disintegrate boundaries (no identity, lose-lose) • Boundary fluidity (diversity with tolerance, contained competition, creative pluralism)
Design of Complex Systems	• Government creates (designs) the boundary conditions within which individuals, business, others can create value • Better designing interface between systems, interactions between systems–interfaces for collective action • Perceive and act in new boundary categories (e.g., creating place value in jurisdictional and civic infrastructures)	• Simultaneous hierarchical and horizontal change • Links in society are focal points • Information a main driver (it knows no boundaries) • No difference between inter- and intra-organization • Boundaryless organization design (holistic work, fluid, invisible boundaries) • What values should determine appropriate location of (new) system boundaries?

proaches) are needed (Rosell, 1995). Such approaches will deal at the level of shared values, goals, and interpretations.

Leadership and Power. Applied to *boundary spanning*, leadership is a boundary function, located at the borders where there is a break between parts of the system; the greater the break, the more leeway for acts of leadership (Katz & Kahn, 1978). As boundary conditions and turf arrangements undergo drastic change and interdependence among organizations heightens, executives will have major responsibilities as ambassadors and interpreters of that environment (Sherwood, 1976). Boundary spanning leadership is a differentiated, distributed function comprising multiple relations (task and socioemotional), and two potentially independent roles (gatekeeper and representative) (Friedman & Polodny, 1992). Boundaries are socially constructed, so rather than examine flows across an assumed boundary, leaders must look explicitly at the boundary and the politics of its social construction (Gilmore, 1982). Applied to *boundarylessness*, traditional language used to portray role relationships, leadership, organizational design and the like is outmoded. This is due to the informatization of society, where information is the dominant resource, and its historically sudden dominance has produced a kind of theory crisis (Cleveland, 1993). The boundaryless metaphor calls for viewing boundaries as paths (Dreaschlin et al., 1994), and seeing new (e.g., more symbolic) boundaries that are invisible or unfamiliar to most managers today (Hirschhorn & Gilmore, 1992).

Psychological Properties. Applied to *boundary spanning*, the subjective boundary thesis has three premises: (1) people set up psychological boundaries when they face uncertainty, feel at risk, and need to contain anxiety, (2) psychological boundaries do not always correspond to formal organizational boundaries, and (3) organizations can function well only when their managers draw and maintain appropriate boundaries in their own roles, and between the organization and its environment (Hirschhorn, 1992). If organizational leadership prevents members from making the links (e.g., that enable its members to enter roles to make links with customers), they will retreat from the boundary and focus solely (and inappropriately) on the internal dynamics of corporate life. Applied to *boundarylessness*, O'Hara (1994) correlates the transition to a global information society and the psychodynamics of how people respond in setting and changing boundaries. She believes those who resist seeing that transition respond either with rigidification of boundaries (global neurosis: compete with outsiders, play "win-lose" games, protect information) or with boundary disintegration or boundarylessness (global psychosis: no boundaries, no identity, no solidarity, lose-lose). Those squarely in the midst of the transition are themselves in a state of boundary shifting (uncertainty), which could eventually lead to boundary fluidity (where collaboration, diversity with tolerance, creative pluralism, and contained competition are more the norm).

Design of Complex Systems. Simon imparts some thoughts that help to portray the essence of the design metaphor:

> The natural sciences are concerned with how things are. Design, on the other hand, is concerned with how things ought to be, with devising artifacts to attain goals. . . . [T]he boundary sciences . . . (are) . . . those that govern the means and the task environment. The artificial world is centered precisely on this interface between outer and inner environments; it is concerned with attaining goals by adapting the former to the latter. (Simon, 1969, pp. 131-133)

Applied to *boundary spanning*, design is the perspective that argues that government creates (designs) the boundary conditions–the frameworks and institutions–within which individuals, businesses, and other nongovernmental social groupings can create value (Kirlin, 1996). In design, boundary spanning translates to government perceiving its role as sustaining and enhancing collective capacity to choose and to act; thus the organization-environment interface is one of many possible interfaces for collective action. Another is designing complex functional systems for service delivery, including better design of interfaces between delivery systems like mental health and justice using boundary spanning positions (Steadman, 1992). Applied to *boundarylessness*, design is simultaneous hierarchical and horizontal change, with an emphasis toward developing the horizontal: changing the focal point of intervention to links in society or webs of organizations. A main driver for the changes is information, which knows no limits, observes no boundaries (Cleveland, 1993). Thus the organization-environment tie might simply be seen as another network link which just happens to span the boundaries of what some observers view as separate organizations (e.g., Lincoln, 1982). In boundarylessness, design aims for holistic work and fluid, invisible boundaries. An important question will be what values determine the appropriate location of new boundaries.

In sum, boundary is more the noun "the what" (what is the limit that is being created, perceived, spanned, or changed). Boundary spanning is more the verb "the how" (the activity or movement across, between, or beyond the limits). Boundaryless is more complex, acting both as an adjective (a modifier to describe what a bounded entity like an organization should be like), or a noun (a result of an aggressive form of boundary spanning), or a verb (the activity of breaking down or redefining a boundary). Boundaryless is a poor metaphor for what it seeks to convey, since its underlying intention is not "no boundaries" but "different boundaries," "changing and fluid boundaries," and "new attitudes for human relationship." Boundary spanning is more anchored in preserving traditional boundaries and "going across them," whereas boundaryless is more anchored in redefining existing boundaries, and creating new arenas for legitimate action. Boundary spanning reflects the fact that organizations are almost always referred to in spatial terms (a boundary separates an organization from its environment, and therefore a boundary becomes a thing to be guarded, crossed, or spanned). Boundaryless, by contrast, is presented partially in spatial terms (e.g., break down the walls), and partially in more temporal terms (e.g., speed, learning, relationships, ideas, and meaning making).

APPLICATION OF BOUNDARY THEORY TO SI IN THE HUMAN SERVICES

Can boundary theory become one frame of reference within which we might interpret and advance the theory and practice of SI in the human services–seeing SI as at heart a question of boundaries? This section presents the results of a preliminary analytic exercise to recast selected SI literature into boundary theory as just described. This effort is intended as an intermediate step to see what theoretical questions might be developed for SI in the human services when boundary is the starting point. The idea is that boundary theory provides a fundamental lens through which to probe analysis and action at the heart of SI that ultimately might yield new questions for a next generation of efforts.

Framing Theoretical Questions About Boundary Elements in SI

In the discussion which follows, conceptual literature on SI in the human services is translated into selected descriptive and normative features of boundary theory. In addition to boundary values, key structural and behavioral elements of boundary theory, drawn from an extensive interdisciplinary survey, include types of boundaries in SI, boundary roles, boundary properties, boundary spanning infrastructure, boundary spanning processes (including boundarylessness), and boundary problems (Halley, 1995). As SI is described, preliminarily, according to each element of boundary theory, theoretical questions are posed to form the basis of an emerging research agenda.

(1) *Types of Boundaries in SI.* In the terms of boundary types, SI is concerned with redefining the nature of boundary relationships throughout the human services (e.g., program boundaries that differentiate categories of need and set the terms of service eligibility, state boundaries, disciplinary boundaries, neighborhood boundaries, public-private sector boundaries, boundaries among human service systems, and boundaries that indicate whether a person has one need or many needs). Is there a typology of human service boundaries? What are the key boundaries for what purposes to be attained in SI? What new boundary types are being created or contemplated under various restructuring schemes? What rationale is implicit in the way existing boundaries are drawn? Are other rationales warranted or possible?

(2) *Boundary Values.* The significance of boundaries in SI in the human services is that they are normative–they are the places at which values, often conflicting, are operationalized and pursued. Such values are complex and contradictory, and range from human values of self-sufficiency and empowerment; to administrative values of coordination, seamlessness, and competition; to delivery values of confidentiality and accountability; and to policy and system values of holism, fragmentation, diversity, and coherence. Public entrepreneurship (Kirlin, 1996) offers the premise that how boundaries (e.g., of complex functional systems or of geographic place) are drawn in general and in the human services will say a great deal about whether the resulting differentiation is overly fragmented or richly diverse according to particular values (e.g., of collective choice, quality of life, effectiveness, efficiency, goods and services). He is positing that government (or governance) can be an integrating mechanism. O'Looney (1993), speaking to the premises underlying the design of social service delivery systems, differentiates the neoconservative privatization or purchase-of-service contracts approach from the more liberal goals of experimentation with social service collaboratives, comprehensive planning, and multidisciplinary staffing–each approach aiming to span human service boundaries by individualizing and customizing services to the individual or family unit as consumer but in quite distinct ways. What values are being enacted at human service boundaries, what are competing or conflicting values, and how are those conflicts being addressed? What new values are (or need to be) created at human service boundaries (known and unknown) in an information economy? How are value contradictions identified and addressed at individual, organization, and inter-organization levels? Should human service systems contribute to the quality of life (of individuals and families) and the physical environment of places (e.g., cities, neighborhoods) and with what value orientations?

(3) *SI boundary roles* have been identified in recent human service literature as broker, innovator, and boundary spanner (Edwards & Austin, 1991). Boundary spanning roles pertinent to SI are also characterized with respect to degree of role specialization. For example, Yessian (1995) argues that the human service workforce has relatively few generalists who have roles spanning program categories and who function in ways intended to integrate services on behalf of clients. Hassett and Austin (1997) note that human service workers are accustomed to dealing with narrowly defined issues and regulations, and will experience difficulty adjusting to the greater autonomy and flexibility envisioned at the local level under certain forms of SI. What roles (other than broker and innovator) are appropriate to accomplish what purposes as efforts are made for people to move across or link among a variety of kinds of boundaries (e.g., intra- and inter- and trans-organizational)? What mix of existing roles and new boundary spanning roles is sought? What skills are called for and what knowledge-base is needed? What social psychological features will performing these roles in human service systems of today and tomorrow induce? What are the implications for existing vertical (disciplinary) versus horizontal (cross-disciplinary) career systems? Can existing human service professions (roles) survive as we know them under a system heavily concentrated on delivery services through boundary spanning arrangements? Should they? What are the implications for the various human service professions?

(4) *Boundary Properties in SI*: The interlocking roles required to break through the numerous existing boundaries among human services will need to address a service system frequently described as having boundary properties that are tight, exclusionary, vague, overlapping, uncertain, and fragmented. The boundaries among human service subspecialities, for example, are becoming less well defined, but it does not thereby follow that the boundaries among human service organizations are blurring. Looking at the existing system of human services (nationally or in a particular locale), what are ideal versus actual boundary properties to realize particular goals? What properties are "healthy" for different kinds of human service boundaries (e.g., what balance of differentiation-integration)? What degree of openness to the environment (permeability) versus stability should human service boundaries have? What properties should information evidence as it flows across and creates boundaries? What types of overlap and redundancy are important to build into the human service delivery system to ensure innovation and protection from failure (suppression of error, detection of error)?

(5) What might be regarded as a *boundary spanning infrastructure in SI*

(i.e., the capacity that is built into specific arenas between and among human service boundaries) has, over time, taken the form of Charity Organization Societies (Kagan & Neville, 1993), the Model Cities apparatus (Hassett & Austin, 1997), umbrella coordinating agencies, collocation, standard federal regions, regional governance structures and processes, public-private partnerships, portfolios of foundations supporting or delivering human services in the name of SI, and service delivery networks of varying kinds. How adequate is this boundary spanning infrastructure to various purposes embedded in SI? What infrastructure should be built within the human services, at and among what differentiations, to appropriately link, integrate, and separate the demarcations of difference that numerous human service boundaries produce? How permanent should various infrastructure mechanisms be and what ought to be their core processes? What are the actual and potential effects on existing institutions of efforts taking place in the interstices of the system?

(6) *Boundary spanning processes (including boundarylessness) identified in the SI* literature would include case management, program decentralization, transorganization management, interdepartmental coordination, and single intake systems to name a few. It is also suggested that SI be regarded as an ongoing process of reform rather than a one-time achievement. These and other SI processes are recast, in the anatomy of boundary theory, as constituting explicit efforts (of a unique logical type) at boundary making and change, boundary governance, boundary tools and control mechanisms, and efforts to work across boundaries within or among organizations. Absent in the literature set examined are characterizations of how to address conflicts and competition among existing human service boundaries, or how to build learning into an ongoing effort to redesign the human service delivery system. What range of boundary spanning processes is available and effective to address the matters of boundary making, change, governance, control, conflict, leadership, and learning? How are boundaries to be changed in the human services–what is the change process? How are different types of human service boundaries set and then spanned? What is being changed–the boundaries or the functions they perform? What is the connection between service integration in the human services and boundarylessness in business literature? What does seamless delivery of human services look like from and among different vantages (e.g., client, policy, program, organization, interorganization)?

(7) *Boundary Problems in SI.* Boundary problems (of structure and process) seen in SI in the human services include: fragmentation of integration efforts when, for example, numerous neighborhood SI efforts cause, in aggregate, even greater fragmentation (Hassett & Austin, 1997);

SI as being a euphemism for program expansion (Kagan & Neville, 1993); confidentiality in information sharing when the boundaries are blurred among programs (Hassett & Austin, 1997); and whether and how SI should proceed from a tight, within-discipline (or program category) vantage or a cross-discipline effort or both. If the rapidly changing context we experience today continues into the future, with ever increasing specialization and atomization, what new boundaries will be created in the human service system and how will they be spanned, managed, and administered? Are separate service systems to disappear altogether, to be replaced by one comprehensive menu-driven system based on solutions to problems? What happens when boundaries of regional policy choices do not correspond to existing human service systems bounded within general purpose governments? What happens when consumer problems are the focal point at key boundaries or when the notion of "service" is dropped–how then are problems addressed, how are human problems bounded? What boundaries are essential to preserve? Given the complexity of the system, how can policy learning (guidance, control, and performance evaluation) be systematically incorporated at key boundaries?

CONCLUSIONS AND IMPLICATIONS

Three conclusions are warranted on the basis of the above discussion. (1) SI is a rich interventive-reflective concept with strong, implicit, normative features that are not always taken into account. (2) Using boundary theory as a starting point, SI, as a concept, can be reframed so as to probe fundamental assumptions, at the level of explanatory theory. This exercise yields a different set of questions to develop and assess future SI efforts in the human services–questions that move beyond but build on the fragmentation-integration dichotomy that is so embedded as a focal point in the SI literature. (3) When the SI literature is recast into the terms of boundary theory, multiple perspectives emerge. Boundary, then, is indeed a starting point for problem formulation, understanding, and normative action in SI. It focuses on the limits set in existing conditions and raises questions about what new limits are possible and desirable. A rich discourse can emerge from such a recasting exercise.

Starting points for discussion, analysis, and action are critically important. (The core question of starting point originated in correspondence to the author from John J. Kirlin, University of Southern California, Sacramento.) They do tend to set the terms (quality, scope, robustness) of the conversation or debate. One should not infer from this paper that there exists an implicit recommendation that all future work in SI commence with boundary as "the" starting point. That is simply not so. Values, for example, could be equally foundational, as could choice. Transorganizational systems are starting points in some interorganization theory (e.g., Cummings, 1984). Fragmentation is a starting point in federalism and intergovernmental relations, where it is often judged negatively (e.g., John et al., 1996). Yet, some political processes recognize the benefits and encourage fragmentation, others seek to moderate it (e.g., checks and balances). Irrespective of the goodness of fragmentation, when fragmentation-integration is the starting point in SI, one can, using boundary theory, reframe the SI concept so as to confront and reflect upon the imperatives relating to the pros and cons of how things are divided (how boundaries are drawn) and how they are connected (how boundaries are integrated). By themselves, starting points of either differentiation, fragmentation, and integration, or individuals, are extremely limited and lead to a narrow range of often dysfunctional policy, behaviors, and beliefs (Kirlin, 1996).

The linkage of boundary theory to the practice of human service integration is critical to the re-examination of the fragmentation-integration dichotomy in the human service system. In essence, how good is fragmentation and how good is integration? Is boundary an intermediate tool that can be used to set an agenda for an ongoing "dialogue about design" (Hassett & Austin, 1997) of human service delivery systems, a dialogue which must include numerous other elements (those raised through boundary as a starting point and those raised by other starting points)? Or is boundary a fundamental question, a starting point that is collinear with many other starting points?

A fundamental argument developed in this paper is really that, under conditions where many starting points are possible, whatever the substantive starting point for SI (whether it is "service," or "integration," or "fragmentation," or "neighborhood," or "person"), a critical and fundamental question will be what are the ensuing boundaries: how are services bounded, how is the human service system itself bounded, how are neighborhoods bounded, and so on. The differentiations we make will influence how important questions of integrative effect (e.g., in quality of life and delivery of human services) are ultimately framed, addressed, and assessed.

REFERENCES

Adams, J.S. (1983). The structure and dynamics of behavior in organizational boundary roles. In M. Dunnette (Ed.), *Handbook of industrial and organizational psychology*. New York: John Wiley & Sons.

Agranoff, R. (1991). Human services integration: Past and present challenges in public administration. *Public Administration Review, 51*(6), 533-542.

Argyris, C. (1970). *Intervention theory and method.* Reading, MA: Addison-Wesley.

Bergquist, W. (1993). *The postmodern organization.* San Francisco: Jossey-Bass Publishers.

Briar, S., & Miller, H. (1971). *Problems and issues in social casework.* New York: Columbia University Press.

Caldwell, A.B. (1994, February). Simultaneous multilevel analysis. *American Psychologist*, 144-145.

Cleveland, H. (1993). *Birth of a new world.* San Francisco: Jossey-Bass.

Cummings, T. (1984). Transorganization development. *Research in Organizational Behavior, 6*, 367-422.

Davidson, W., & Davis, S. (1990). Management and organization principles for the information economy. *Human Resource Management, 29*, 365-383.

Devanna, M.A., & Tichey, N. (1990). Creating the competitive organization of the 21st Century: The boundaryless corporation. *Human Resource Management, 29*, 455-71.

Dreaschlin, J., Kobrinski, E., & Passen, A. (1994). The boundary path of exchange: A new metaphor for leadership. *Leadership and Organization Development Journal, 15*(6), 16-23.

Edwards, R.L., & Austin, D. (1991). Managing effectively in an environment of competing values. In R.L. Edwards & J.A. Yankey (Eds.), *Skills for effective human services management.* Silver Spring, MD: National Association of Social Workers.

Friedman, R.A., & Polodny, J. (1992). Differentiation of boundary spanning roles: Labor negotiations and implications for role conflict. *Administrative Science Quarterly, 37*, 28-47.

Gell-Mann, M. (1994). *The Quark and the Jaguar: Adventures in the Simple and the Complex.* NY: W.H. Freeman and Company.

Gilmore, T. (1982). Leadership and boundary management. *Journal of Applied Behavioral Science, 18*, 343-356.

Halley, A.A. (1995). *Toward a formal concept of boundary: Testing emerging theory against two public administration cases.* Unpublished doctoral dissertation, University of Southern California.

Hassett, S., & Austin, M.J. (1997). Service integration: Something old and something new. *Administration in Social Work*, Special Issue on Integrative Services, *21*(3/4).

Hirschhorn, L. (1992). *The workplace within: Psychodynamics of organizational life.* Cambridge, MA: The MIT Press.

Hirschhorn, L., & Gilmore, T. (1992). The new boundaries of the boundaryless company. *Harvard Business Review, 70*, 104-115.

John, D., Halley, A.A., & Fosler, S. (1996). Remapping federalism: The rediscovery of civic governance. In J.S. Jun & D.S. Wright (Eds.), *Globalization and decentralization: Institutional contexts, policy issues, and intergovernmental relations in Japan and the United States.* Washington, DC: Georgetown University Press.

Johnston, D.M. (1988). *The theory and history of ocean boundary-making*. Kingston and Montreal: McGill-Queen's University Press.
Kagan, S.L. with Neville, P. (1993). *Integrating services for children and families: Understanding the past to shape the future*. New Haven, CT: Yale University Press.
Katz, D., & Kahn, R. (1978). *The Social Psychology of Organizations (2nd ed.)*. New York: John Wiley & Sons.
Kirlin, J. (1994). Emerging regional organizational and institutional forms: Strategies and prospects for transcending localism. Washington, DC: National Academy of Public Administration, NAPA-NIRA Conference. (Published May, 1996, by Georgetown University Press.)
Kirlin, J. (1996, January). What government must do well: Creating value for society. *Journal of Public Administration Research and Theory*.
Landau, M. (1969, July/August). Redundancy, rationality, and the problem of duplication and overlap. *Public Administration Review*, 346-358.
Leifer, R., & Huber, G. (1977). Relations among perceived environmental uncertainty, organizational structure, and boundary spanning behavior. *Administrative Science Quarterly, 22*, 235-247.
Lincoln, J.R. (1982). Intra- and inter-organizational networks. *Research in the Sociology of Organizations, 1*, 1-38.
Martin, P. et al. (1983). The concept of integrated services reconsidered. *Social Science Quarterly 64*(4), 747-763.
Michael, D. (1995). What now? Some reflections on the context and conditions for learning. In D. Michael (Ed.), *On learning to plan and planning to learn*. Alexandria, VA: Miles River Press.
Miles, R. (1980). *Macro organizational behavior*. Glenview, IL: Scott, Foresman and Company.
Moore, S. (1992). Case management and the integration of services: How service delivery systems shape case management. *Social Work, 37*(5), 418-423.
O'Hara, M. (1994). Future mind: Is humanity headed for psychic breakdown or consciousness breakthrough in an era of globalization? Unpublished manuscript. Meridian International Institute, San Francisco.
O'Looney, J. (1993). Beyond privatization and service integration: Organizational models for service delivery. *Social Service Review, 67*(1), 501-534.
Robertson, P.J. (1995). Involvement in boundary spanning activity: Mitigating the relationship between work setting and behavior. *Journal of Public Administration Research and Theory, 5*(1), 73-98.
Rosell, S. (1995). *Changing maps: Governing in a world of rapid change*. Ottawa: Carleton University Press.
Schon, D. (1971). *Beyond the stable state*. New York: W.W. Norton & Company.
Sherwood, F.P. (1976). The American Public Executive in the Third Century. *Public Administration Review*, 586-591.
Simon, H. (1969). *The sciences of the artificial (2nd ed)*. Cambridge, MA: The MIT Press.
Steadman, H.J. (1992). Boundary spanners: A key component for effective inter-

actions of the justice and mental health systems. *Law and Human Behavior, 16*(1), 75-87.

Thompson, J.D. (1967). *Organizations in action: Social science bases of administrative theory.* New York: McGraw Hill Book Company.

Tushman, M. (1977). Special boundary roles in the innovation process. *Administrative Science Quarterly 22*, 587-605.

Weinberg, G.M. (1975). *An introduction to general systems thinking.* New York: John Wiley & Sons.

Weiner, M. (1990). *Human services management: Analysis and applications.* Belmont, CA: Wadsworth Publishing Company.

Yessian, M. (1995). Learning from experience: Integrating human services. *Public Welfare, 53*(3), 34-39.

Index

